D0415377

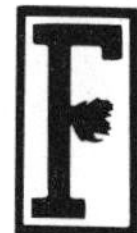

ALSO BY ARNIE BAKER, M.D.

SMART CYCLING—SUCCESSFUL TRAINING & RACING FOR RIDERS OF ALL LEVELS

THE ESSENTIAL CYCLIST

BICYCLING MEDICINE

Cycling Nutrition, Physiology, and Injury Prevention and Treatment for Riders of All Levels

Arnie Baker, M.D.

A FIRESIDE BOOK

Published by Simon & Schuster

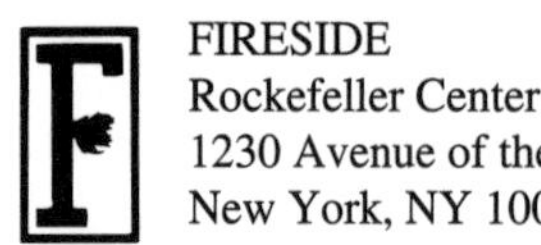

FIRESIDE
Rockefeller Center
1230 Avenue of the Americas
New York, NY 10020

Designed by Pagesetters/IPA

Manufactured in the United States of America

10 9 8 7

Library of Congress Cataloging-in-Publication Data

Baker, Arnie.
Bicycling medicine : cycling nutrition, physiology, and injury prevention and treatment for riders of all levels / Arnie Baker.
p. cm.
Previously published in 1995 with subtitle: Cycling health, fitness & injury explained : for riders & racers of all levels.
Includes bibliographical references and index.
1. Cycling—Health aspects. 2. Cycling—Physiological aspects. 3. Cycling accidents. I. Title
RC1220.C8B36 1998
617.1'027—dc21

98-27500
CIP

ISBN 0-684-84443-5 (alk. paper)

The author has used his best efforts in preparing this book and the information contained herein. These efforts include a review of medical literature and the development, research, and testing of theories, treatments, and programs to determine their effectiveness.

The author makes no warranty of any kind, expressed or implied, with regard to the information contained in this book.

The author shall not be liable in the event of incidental or consequential damages in connection with, or arising out of, the furnishing, performance, or use of information, associated instructions, programs, and/or claims of results or productivity gains.

This book describes common situations and common treatments. Generalizations or applicability of information contained in this book may not apply to any specific individual. Individual conditions may appear to be similar to descriptions in this book, but in fact may be different conditions. Different treatments may apply. Although pain and other problems in athletes are often attributable to exercise, it is a mistake to so assume.

All readers are especially cautioned to obtain medical consultation in the event of any medical problems.

All readers are especially cautioned to consider obtaining medical consultation before entering into any athletic training program.

Trademarked names appear throughout this book. The names and entities that own the trademarks are not listed. Trademark symbols may not always appear. The publisher states that it is using the names only for editorial purposes and to the benefit of the trademark owner, with no intention of infringing upon that trademark.

Acknowledgments

I have been helped by many people, not only in the specific preparation of this book but also in my development as a physician, coach, and racer.

I thank Barbara Baker, my first patient; Dr. Huntington Sheldon, for teaching me to question conventional wisdom; Dr. Abe Mayman, for teaching me about the office practice of medicine; Dr. Sid Feldman, for teaching me about being a mensch; Dr. Leon Speroff, for showing me the value of organization in the presentation of information. Of course, my father, for making me feel guilty about being anything but a physician, and then being so proud when I became one.

I thank Barbara Baker and Brian Begley, who proofread the first self-published edition; Mike Schnorr, for illustrations; Dean Golich, for reviewing the physiology section; Dr. John Morse, for cardiology advice; and Gero McGuffin, who not only has helped in proofing and criticism but rides with me every day.

Contents

Part Two:

Physiology

Part Three:

General Prevention and Treatment of Injuries

Part Five:

General Health

Introduction

This book is about health, fitness, and injury in bicyclists. It is a response to the questions and problems cyclists have approached me with in my practice as a physician, cyclist, racer, coach, and consultant over the last fifteen years.

In cycling, as in any sport, if you can accurately understand how your body works—how it gets nourished and how it responds to training, injury, and disease—you may be able to use that knowledge to help your body perform better.

For example, almost all cyclists I've met are concerned about nutrition, but many lack an accurate factual knowledge of nutrition principles. The first part of *Bicycling Medicine* will provide readers with knowledge about health through good nutrition. This part may also provide a basis for developing important habits not only for cycling but for health in general.

Many fitness and racer cyclists are very interested in the physiology of cycling; they want to know how being active affects their bodies. The important exercise physiology issues facing bicyclists are discussed in the second part.

Prevention of injury is possible. Prevention means, for example, finding the right bicycle and fitting it properly. Nonetheless, injuries do occur. In the third part, in addition to prevention, the options and general principles of injury treatment, without reference to any specific injury, are discussed.

Bicycling-related injury and medical problems can affect almost any part of the body. Almost all of the bicycling-related problems that cyclists have are examined in the fourth part. Self-diagnosis and treatment may be possible with the information presented in this part, but please be cautious. The information given is by no means a substitute for professional consultation. For any persistent or potentially serious injuries you are urged to seek professional help. Besides helping you decide when an injury requires professional treatment, this part may help you understand the treatment you receive.

In addition to specific ones, cyclists frequently suffer from more generalized problems that can affect their performance, such as fatigue, interrupted sleep, and a host of non–cycling-related illnesses. Medication may also affect performance. Even though many of these conditions may not be caused by cycling, they have important ramifications for the cyclist, and so are discussed in part five.

This book does contain some information about bicycling training and racing. Much more detail concerning these aspects of bicycling can be found in my companion book, *Smart Cycling*.

A Note Before You Begin

Plus ça change, plus c'est la même chose. (The more things change, the more they are the same thing.)

—Karr

I've tried to present the best information available. There is no *one* theory; there is no *one* right way; there are no absolutes. To see what I mean, consider the following examples:

Exercise

Those of you reading this book who enjoy exercising may find it difficult to believe: During certain eras, exercise was thought to be dangerous for health. For example, the ancient Greeks' love for sports brought it to the highest levels, yet Hippocrates and Galen believed that competition in the sports arena brought an early death. The Surgeon General of the U.S. Navy wrote in 1911 that rigorous training for physical sports was dangerous to health.

Nutrition

In the fifties when I was growing up, I was told that eggs were the perfect food. They contain good protein and are an excellent source of vitamins and minerals. Thirty years later I learned that my mother was wrong and that a single egg could ruin a whole week for cholesterol intake—cholesterol was bad. Still later, in the early nineties, I learned that the importance of maintaining low cholesterol levels had been overstated and that treatment for high cholesterol might be counterproductive, since the medications were said to cause many side effects, especially in the elderly. Now, in the late nineties, medication is again in, but dietary fat, rather than egg cholesterol, is said to be the villain. As I was growing up I learned that some fat in the diet made food taste good. Later I learned that fat was harmful, a cause of heart disease and cancer, and that it should ideally be severely limited in the diet. I also learned that fat decreases athletic performance. Later I read that people get too little of the right fats and that an increase would improve athletic performance.

Physiology

Altitude training (training at elevations over 7,000 feet) as a method of performance enhancement has, at various times, been seen as a panacea for improvement. We now think that if altitude training is timed correctly, it *can* help certain aerobic sports—but at the same time, it *can* be harmful. Although some physiological gains can be made, some are restricted.

There are many theories about training. Should base miles and strength work form the basis of off-season training, with interval work added during the racing season? Or should intervals be maintained year round, and endurance added only when needed? Most coaches and physiologists favor the first approach, but there is debate.

At one time cyclists used to just ride lots of miles to improve fitness. Then came an age of *quality* miles. Yet, more recent studies have shown that all things being equal, quantity of training is one of the most important predictors of performance. Who would have thought that the hour distance record (set by Chris Boardman in 1996) would come from training lots of miles below race pace, rather than quality miles at pace?

Medical Treatment

Should scabs be allowed to form over wounds to protect them? I don't think so—healing is much faster and scarring is less when their formation is prevented—but not everyone agrees with me.

The Best We Know Now

So, as you can see, some concepts about bicycling medicine, health, fitness, and injuries change; some issues remain controversial. This book attempts to provide the best current information available.

Part One

DIET AND NUTRITION

The known principles of sound diet and nutrition help ensure optimal performance. Consistent attention to nutrition helps the athlete perform to genetic potential.

Nutrition—The Big Picture

The major requirements of sound nutrition are water, calories, vitamins, and minerals. Calories come from carbohydrates, proteins, and fats. All known caloric, protein, vitamin, and mineral needs can be met by a varied and healthful diet.

The body needs a certain amount of protein and fat to work properly, but the necessary amounts are small compared with the amounts most of us consume. Almost all of us who eat meat, fish, fowl, or dairy products regularly get more than enough protein; we don't have to monitor our intake. The same situation applies to fat intake, whether you're a vegetarian or not: most of us get many times the daily requirement of fat.

Since carbohydrates are inexpensive, easily digested and metabolized, and associated with less health risk than fats, they form the dietary cornerstone of caloric intake. Also, fortunately, as you'll read soon, they are the preferred fuel for high-intensity exercise and the mainstay of the aerobic endurance athlete.

The needs of a cyclist may, at times, differ from the nutrition required for good health in general, but this is unusual. General nutrition principles still apply. A variety of foodstuffs in moderation provide a "balanced diet."

In some ways, optimum nutrition is a lot like a bicycle tire—you need the right amount of air. Too little and your tire is flat; you don't go fast enough. Too much and it may have side effects: a harsh ride or a burst.

Not enough of the right nutrients, and you may fatigue easily. Too much, and side effects may also limit your performance!

The USDA Food Pyramid

Figure 1-1

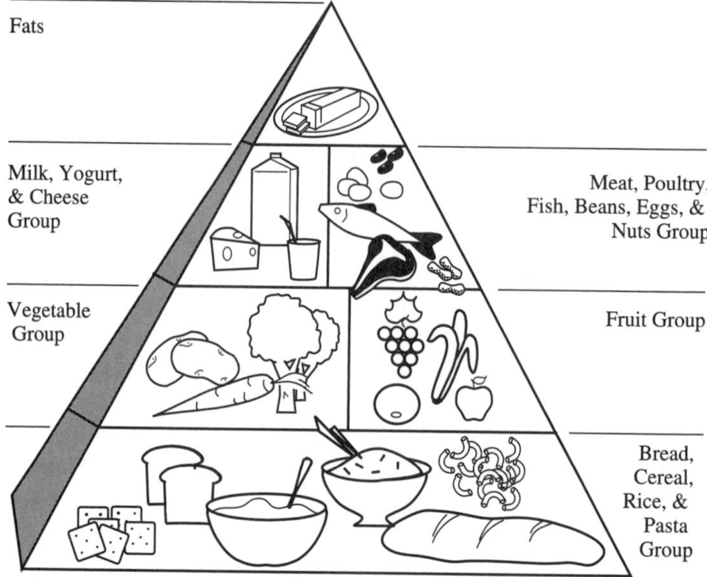

The USDA food pyramid

Counting Servings

The U.S. Department of Agriculture food pyramid shows that the majority of foods you eat should come from the base: the bread, cereal, rice and pasta group. Potatoes are also in this group. Six to eleven servings a day are recommended. Two to four servings of vegetables and two to four servings of fruit are recommended daily. Two to three servings of fat-free milk, yogurt, or cheese and two to three servings of meat, poultry, fish, beans, eggs, or nuts are recommended daily. Fats, oils, and sweets are to be used only sparingly.

Counting Servings—Not

Most people do not want or need to go through life counting portions of food. The basic principle is that most of your calories should come from starches: bread, cereals, rice or pasta. Fruits and vegetables are good for you. Fatty foods and whole milk or cream products are too fatty to be considered healthy choices. Almost all foods now have labels that list serving sizes, calories per serving, and calories from fat.

Caloric Nutrients

Calories provide the energy that the body needs to operate. The major nutrient divisions of carbohydrate, protein, and fat can all be used by the body to provide energy. (Alcohol also provides calories.)

An aerobic endurance athlete may require 8 to 10 grams per kilogram of body weight per day of carbohydrate and 1.5 grams per kilogram per day of protein. Meeting these requirements is more important than giving a percentage formula. However, percentage formulas are easier for some people to understand: 60% to 70% of calories might come from carbohydrates, 10% to 20% from protein, 20% to 25% from fat. On the basis of current information, such a diet not only is optimal for athletes but is probably the most healthful diet for the general population as well.

Protein and carbohydrate supply 4 calories of energy for each gram. Fat supplies 9 calories for each gram. A pound of carbohydrate provides less than one-half the calories of a pound of fat. It has less than one-half the caloric density of fat.

Caloric foods not promptly used for immediate energy are converted to glycogen or stored as fats. Normally, up to 2,000 calories are stored as glycogen; and normally, in excess of 50,000 calories are stored as fat.

Excess calories may lead to weight gain, which is detrimental to health and performance. The major nutritional health problem in the United States today is *overnutrition.*

Although obesity is a serious problem, so is undernutrition. Many athletes whose performance depends on low body weight are subject to illness because they are too thin. This is discussed further in "Too Thin?" in the women's health chapter on page 269.

Body fat testing and guidelines for health and performance are discussed in "Measuring Body Fat" on page120.

Carbohydrates

Carbohydrates are simple sugars; complex sugars, or starches; and indigestible sugars, or fiber.

SIMPLE SUGARS

Simple sugars are categorized as single- or double-molecule sugars. *Single-molecule* sugars include glucose, fructose, and galactose. *Double-molecule* sugars include sucrose (table sugar), lactose (milk sugar), and maltose (malt sugar).

Refined sugars are processed sugars devoid of other nutrients. *Natural* simple sugars, found in fruits, juices, milk, and vegetables are associated with vitamins and minerals.

Simple sugars are the building blocks of complex sugars, or starches.

Foods with a lot of simple sugars or simple carbohydrates are often sweet. They include candies, fruit, and nondiet soft drinks. Simple sugars usually come with few vitamins or minerals and are therefore often referred to as "empty calories."

COMPLEX SUGARS—STARCHES

When simple sugars form long chains of carbohydrates, they are called "complex." Complex carbohydrates, or starches, are often associated with other nutrients. Foods consisting primarily of complex carbohydrates are pasta, breads, potatoes, and grains. Ingested complex carbohydrates are digested (broken down) into simple sugars before being absorbed into the bloodstream.

The body re-forms a complex carbohydrate for energy storage called glycogen. Glycogen is the critical fuel for performance in the high aerobic and anaerobic threshold range, and is stored primarily within muscle cells and the liver. When one exercises for a couple of hours at high intensity, it's easy to use up these stores.

Since complex carbohydrates are associated with other nutrients and are critical for glycogen replacement, they form the cornerstone of meal planning.

Maltodextrins or *glucose polymers* are medium-length chained carbohydrates, partially broken down from naturally occurring complex carbohydrates. They are often found in "energy bars." The contention that they provide a more constant source of energy than simple sugars, one that is easier to digest than naturally occurring complex carbohydrates, is only partially true. The discussion of glycemic index, below, explains why.

Fiber is indigestible complex carbohydrate. Fiber plays a role in overall health but has little bearing on athletic performance.

GLYCEMIC INDEX

It used to be thought that simple sugars entered the bloodstream rapidly but that their effects on energy production were short-lived. It used to be thought that complex sugars provided a steadier release of food energy.

Studies have shown that the rate of release of sugar into the bloodstream, or glycemic effect, is related to factors other than whether sugars are simple or complex. The rate of digestion of sugars has more to do with cooking, ripening, and the presence of fiber, fats, and proteins associated with the sugar than it does with the presence of simple sugars. For example, a well-baked potato releases sugar into the bloodstream almost as rapidly as glucose. The release of simple sugars in whole milk is delayed by the presence of fat. Bananas release sugar more rapidly when ripe. Simple sugars consumed as part of a meal raise blood sugar more slowly than when consumed by themselves.

Pure glucose is assigned a glycemic index of 100. The rate of release of sugar into the bloodstream caused by other substances is compared with the release rate of pure glucose.

Sugars that have a glycemic index greater than 80 are considered to be released quickly. Sugars that have a glycemic index between 40 and 80 are considered to be released moderately. Sugars with a glycemic index below 40 are released slowly.

Sugars that release quickly and help to spare or replace burned glycogen may be suitable during or after exercise. Sugars that release moderately slowly may be more suitable several hours before or after exercise.

Table 1-1 **Glycemic Index of Foods**

Glucose	100	Bananas	60	Ice cream	36
Potato, baked	98	Sucrose	60	Milk, whole	34
Carrots, cooked	92	Pasta	50	Milk, fat free	32
Honey	87	Potato chips	50	Beans, kidney	30
Cornflakes	83	Oatmeal	50	Lentils	30
Rice	72	Orange juice	50	Fructose	20
Bread	70	Oranges	43	Carrots, raw	16
Candy bars	65	Beans, baked	40	Beans, soy	15
Raisins	65	Apples	40	Peanuts	10

Protein

Proteins are important in muscle structure and metabolism. Amino acids are the building blocks of proteins. The body can make some of these amino acids, but some must be obtained through the diet. These are called essential amino acids.

Protein is needed for muscle formation. Proteins are also used to transport other chemicals in the bloodstream. Enzymes, which are proteins, are important in speeding up many body processes.

Foods that contain all the "essential" amino acids are called "complete proteins." Foods that contain only some amino acids are "incomplete" proteins.

Foods rich in proteins are meat, fish, fowl, and milk products.

Vegetarians may sometimes have difficulty in obtaining enough high-quality protein. Nuts, grains, and legumes have incomplete proteins. If eaten together, or within the same day, they may complement one another, providing all the essential amino acids.

The U.S. Recommended Daily Allowance (RDA) of protein is 45 to 63 grams for men and 44 to 50 grams for women. Needs may be increased for people who are weight training. The maximum amount of protein bodybuilders require is 1 gram per pound of body weight.

Proteins, when used by the body for energy, are expensive. They cost more than carbohydrates. Expensive protein supplements are usually a waste of money.

Fats

Fats are primarily triglycerides, the major storage form of calories. Triglycerides have a glycerol backbone, to which are attached three fatty acid chains. Fats make foods calorically dense. A 4-ounce portion of oil has about 1,000 calories, but 4 ounces of carrots, celery, apples, or lettuce have less than 50 calories.

Fats taste good to most of us—they make carbohydrates more palatable. They are also relatively inexpensive.

A small amount of fat is necessary in the diet. Diets that derive more than 30% of their calories from fat are considered unhealthy, because excess dietary fat is associated with obesity, heart disease, stroke, and some cancers.

Fats that are liquid at room temperature are referred to as oils.

Polyunsaturated fats (fats with more than one chemical "double-bond"—potential sites for hydrogen binding) are believed to be better for health than saturated or hydrogenated fats. Polyunsaturated fats tend to be softer or liquid at room temperature rather than firm or solid. Diets that derive more than 10% of their calories from saturated fat are considered unhealthy.

Fats (especially) and proteins slow the workings of the stomach and intestines in comparison with carbohydrates. By analogy, one might say that high-glycemic carbohydrates are like burning paper, medium- and low-glycemic carbohydrates are like burning wood, and fats are like burning coal.

Slow long-distance cycling burns mostly fats. Higher-intensity efforts require not only fats but the higher levels of energy provided by glycogen.

Although fats are the fuel that supply the most calories during physical activity, that energy need not come from ingested fats. Remember that all caloric foods—carbohydrates, fats, and proteins—not promptly used for energy or stored as glycogen are metabolized and stored as fats.

Diet: Why High Carbohydrates?

Calories come from carbohydrates, proteins, and fats. Complex carbohydrates formed the backbone of athletes' diets from the sixties through the eighties as research demonstrating their value flourished.

Some challenges to high-carbohydrate diets have surfaced in recent years. The so-called 40-30-30 ratio of carbohydrates, proteins, and fats has become popular with many.

What is the basis for the more traditional endurance aerobic athlete 65-15-20 diet, and should we stick with it?

What We're Talking About

The traditional high-performance aerobic-endurance diet consists of 60% to 70% of calories as carbohydrates, 10% to 15% as protein, and 15% to 20% as fat. Studies have shown that such a diet is typical of Tour-de-France riders. This has been referred to as a high-carbohydrate diet.

Recent articles in bicycling and triathlon magazines have noted the "diet revolution": a 40-30-30 diet, in which carbohydrates make up only 40% of total calories, and proteins and fats make up the divided remainder.

Some have referred to this diet as "high fat." In terms of percentage fat content, it is typical of the average North American diet. However, it has a higher than average protein content.

Where Energy Comes From

Carbohydrates, proteins, and fats can all be used to make energy. Approximately 4 calories are produced from each gram of carbohydrate or protein metabolized; about 9 calories are produced from each gram of fat.

Where Energy Goes

The body needs energy to keep the brain working, the heart pumping, the kidneys filtering blood. The amount of energy needed for basal metabolic activities depends on the size of the individual—but let's say the average is about 1,000 calories per day.

The body also needs energy for physical activities—everything from light activity such as walking to the heavy activity of high-end endurance exercise. Heavy activity can use several thousand calories a day.

Food energy that the body doesn't need doesn't evaporate. The body does not excrete calories. All calories ingested are either used to produce energy or stored as fat. Excess carbohydrates and protein are converted to fat and stored along with the excess dietary fat in the body's fat deposits. (Importantly, the reverse does not happen except to a very minor degree—only a small portion of fats can be converted back to carbohydrates.)

How the Body Makes Energy

The body uses fat, carbohydrates, and protein to make energy via partially different metabolic pathways. Protein is usually used in building muscle or other functions; its contribution to energy production is small and will be ignored in this discussion.

At rest and at low levels of activity, relatively more fat is used for energy production. As activity levels become more intense, more carbohydrate is used to make energy.

Fat requires relatively more oxygen to burn than carbohydrate. Although fat contributes to energy production during exercise, carbohydrate is the key to high efforts. Once your heart rate climbs over 75% of your maximum, more than 50% of your energy is coming from carbohydrate. (To learn more about maximum heart rate, read "Heart Rate Training" on page 75.)

Traditionally, the amount of carbohydrate energy used was believed to be higher than that shown in Table 1-2. The amount of carbohydrate metabolism was originally calculated on the basis of respiratory exchange ratios determined from the relative concentrations of carbon dioxide and oxygen expired. Newer analysis techniques have suggested that fat contribution is greater than was previously thought. This subject is discussed in more depth in the next chapter, "Energy Sources at Various Exercise Levels."

Table 1-2

Heart Rate % of Maximum	Carbohydrate Energy %
65	15
75	50
85	60
90	70

Percent contribution of carbohydrates to energy metabolism at selected percentages of maximum heart rate.

Glycogen Is Crucial for High-End Energy

The body has about 2,000 calories of carbohydrates stored for energy. This stored carbohydrate, or glycogen, is found in the liver and in muscle.

Normally, about 50,000 calories of energy are stored as fat. But fat calories can be used only for moderate energy level production at most. A one-hour time trial uses up almost all the glycogen stored in muscle. It's easy for a high-performance athlete to burn up almost all stored glycogen with a day's workout. It's glycogen replacement we need for repeated day-after-day training. Glycogen exhaustion limits the role of stored carbohydrates in very long-distance endurance activities that take most of a day or longer to complete.

Performance Time Related to Glycogen

There is a direct relationship between the amount of time a fit individual can perform anaerobic-threshold level work and the amount of glycogen present. The more glycogen initially present, the longer an individual can maintain an anaerobic threshold level effort.

The graph in Figure 1-2 demonstrates this linear relationship. A well-rested, recovered athlete has 100% of normal muscle glycogen. Prior exercise or not replacing carbohydrates results in lower levels. It is possible for muscle to have more than a "normal" amount of glycogen through a process known as glycogen loading, described below.

Figure 1-2

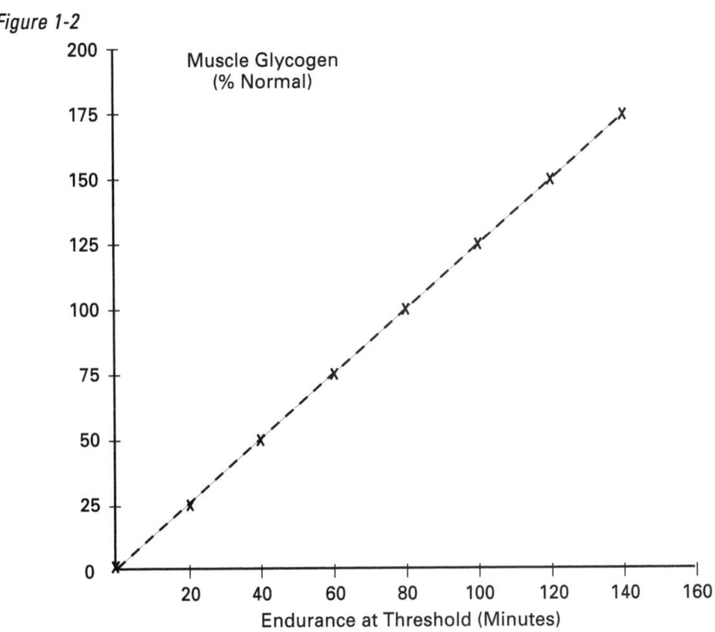

Endurance at threshold is directly correlated with glycogen stores in muscle prior to exercise.

A Lot of Carbohydrates Are Needed

Do some very rough arithmetic. A 130-pound female bicycle racer might use 800 calories in basal metabolism and 2,200 in training or racing. Of those 2,200 calories, 200 might come from fat and 2,000 from glycogen for high-energy use. All that glycogen needs to be replaced in order for the bicycle racer to work as hard the next day. To make the figures simple, and use some basic assumptions, 2,000 out of 3,000 calories is two-thirds, or 66%, of caloric needs. If only 40% of her calories consumed that day come from carbohydrates, full glycogen replacement will not be achieved.

Glycogen Exhaustion

Repeated bouts of moderate- or high-intensity endurance work can quickly exhaust glycogen reserves. Figure 1-3 shows what happens.

A daily program of two hours of activity leads to reduced glycogen levels. Glycogen levels are maintained in proportion to the amount of carbohydrates ingested. Glycogen exhaustion occurs quickly unless a high-carbohydrate diet is maintained. On the morning after three days of heavy endurance training, an athlete consuming a 70% carbohydrate diet still has about 75% of normal glycogen levels. An athlete consuming a 40% carbohydrate diet has less than 15% of normal levels.

Glycogen Loading

Increased glycogen stores can be created through what is called glycogen loading. This involves a period of (1) glycogen use or exhaustion with heavy exercise, followed by (2) reduced activity accompanied by a high-carbohydrate diet. (Athletes also used to consume a high-fat diet in the first period, but further studies have shown that there is no need to incorporate this strategy to successfully load glycogen.)

Riding Slow to Burn Fat—Not!

There is a popular misconception that in order to lose weight, i.e., fat, one needs to ride slowly, at a low aerobic training pace.

It is true that a greater percentage of the calories burned during exercise at lower intensities comes from fat. But fat calories are also burned during resting or basal metabolic activities. If your training time is limited, you'll lose about as much fat by riding at a higher intensity. Further, high-intensity training stimulates the body to burn more fat after exercise is ended, and it also gets you into better shape.

In order for you to lose weight, your net daily caloric expenditure must ex-

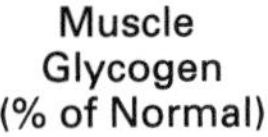

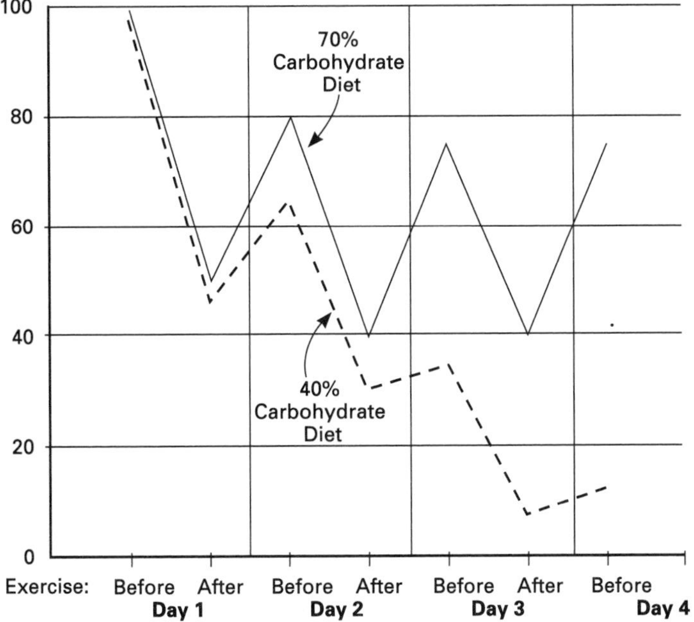

Progressive depletion of glycogen stores after three days of two-hour bouts of heavy endurance training with either 40% or 70% carbohydrate diet.

ceed your intake. To lose one pound of fat, you've got to have a deficit of 3,500 calories. So, in order to lose one pound a week, you've got to use 500 more calories daily than you take in.

If your basal metabolic need is 1,000 calories a day, your daily caloric deficit (say, 500 calories)—and weight loss—can be met with basal fat calories just as easily as your exercise calories.

A relevant diet question is this: Do those calories come at the expense of glycogen or fat stores?

If you have relatively unlimited time, a day with a four-hour low-intensity ride will burn the same number of calories as a day with a two-hour high-intensity ride: 3,000 total calories—2,000 calories for the activity and 1,000 calories for basal metabolism. If you do this every day of the week, and if you ingest just 2,500 calories, the deficit of 500 calories will contribute to an average weight loss of one pound a week. If you have only two hours, you'll burn fewer calories with low-intensity work than with high-intensity work. And with a caloric surplus of 500, you'll *gain* an average of a pound a week.

Table 1-3

Calories Used	65% Max HR 2 Hours	65% Max HR 4 Hours	85% Max HR 2 Hours
Daily basal: Fat	1,000	1,000	1,000
Exercise	1,000	2,000	2,000
Glycogen	150	300	1,200
Fat	850	1,700	800
Daily total: Fat	1,850	2,700	1,800
Daily total: Glycogen and fat	2,000	3,000	3,000

Daily basal and exercise calories used during exercise of selected duration and intensity. Max HR: maximum heart rate.

A 2,500-calorie diet that is 65% carbohydrates will provide 1,625 calories toward glycogen replacement. A 40% carbohydrate diet will provide only 1,000 calories of carbohydrate.

If you eat a high-carbohydrate diet, you will be able to better replace your glycogen, and you will be able to train day after day. If you don't, your glycogen tank won't be filled. After a few days you won't be able to train at as high an intensity level, and you'll run out of high-performance energy—glycogen. You'll have to train more slowly and longer to lose as much fat.

The moral is this: if your time is limited, within the limits of your overall training program, ride hard and eat a high-carbohydrate diet.

What Do Scientific Studies Show?

If you look at scientific research, you've got to look at research designed to answer the right questions.

Are you a RAAM rider looking to improve fat metabolism? Are you a weekend warrior? Are you a recreational rider, riding a few times a week at no more than 75% of your maximum heart rate? Are you a frequent high-end training and racing athlete?

The literature supporting high-carbohydrate diets for high-end aerobic endurance athletes is massive, international, and accepted. The literature supporting higher-fat diets is small. The only study I was able to find concerned athletes who consumed a nighttime meal of high (45%) fat vs. low (20%) fat the night before a cycling ergometer test. The riders were rested, were not subject to previous glycogen depletion, and had no breakfast.

40-30-30 proponents often quote this study, saying that it shows the superiority of increasing fat in the athlete's diet. One could just as easily say it supports the notion of eating breakfast!

Diet and Health

The current medical wisdom is that reducing fat in our diets is important for general health. It is believed that fat contributes to heart disease and cancer. Fortunately, the high-carbohydrate diet for athletes reduces fat.

Insulin and High-Carbohydrate Diets

Proponents of a higher fat diet (for example, the 40-30-30 diet) point to diabetes and "carbohydrate poisoning." They claim that high loads of carbohydrates are associated with high insulin levels. They say that insulin contributes to the conversion of carbohydrate to fat, and that increased fat stores contribute to insulin resistance and diabetes. Therefore, so the argument goes, we should reduce our intake of carbohydrates.

I partially agree. But insulin also increases the formation of glycogen. And not all carbohydrates cause a rapid rise in insulin levels. The glycemic index—the degree to which foodstuffs increase blood sugar—is variable for different carbohydrates. Complex carbohydrates are the mainstay of the American Diabetes Association's dietary recommendations.

Moreover, the body's insulin response to sugar load during exercise is effectively turned off by the body's secretion of catecholamines (adrenaline and related compounds). Although carbohydrates consumed before exercise do increase insulin levels, they still result in improved performance.

Pre-, During- and Post-Activity Feeding

The athlete can divide calorie intake into two areas: calories in and around the training or racing period, and all the rest.

Fats delay the emptying of the stomach. When blood supplies are diverted to the intestines to aid digestion, less blood is available to go to the working muscles. Consequently, big meals and fatty meals ingested within an hour of intense exercise can cause performance problems.

Carbohydrate consumption immediately before or during training or racing can spare glycogen and allow high-end energy production to be maintained longer. Carbohydrate replacement within a couple of hours, preferably as soon as possible after exercise, can help "refuel the glycogen tank" more effectively, allowing repeated training within a shorter period of time.

Caveats

If you have an extra twenty-four hours' recovery before your next high-performance aerobic-endurance ride—i.e., a rest day—you've got a lot more time to replace your glycogen, so a reduced carbohydrate, higher-fat diet is not going to worsen your performance.

If you're entering a road race of 70 miles and it's not going to get "hot and heavy" until two hours or 50 miles into the race, a balanced meal not based solely on carbohydrate may stay with you longer, keeping up your energy stores longer. Tour de France riders, for example, typically include some fats and protein along with their pre-race carbohydrate meals.

If you're not going to eat the morning of a ride, an evening meal with a high fat content may actually help, because your sleeping glycogen stores may be spared by the slower digestion and metabolism of fats.

Bottom Line

Aerobic endurance athletes need 6 to 10 grams of carbohydrates per kilogram (3 to 5 grams per pound) of body weight per day to replace or top up glycogen stores. They need about 1.5 grams per kilogram (0.7 grams per pound) of protein.

There is no point in consuming a diet higher in fat to spare glycogen if the net result is that you have less glycogen to spare.

Energy Sources at Various Exercise Levels

Energy for exercising muscle comes from fat, carbohydrate, and protein. Fat energy may come from the bloodstream by way of adipose tissue or the intestine, or from fat stores in muscle.

Carbohydrates may come from blood sugar (from the liver by way of stored glycogen or metabolized amino acids, or from the intestine by the absorption of carbohydrates) or from glycogen stores in muscle. About 2,500 calories of intramuscular fat (triglyceride) energy are stored in muscle cells—more than the 1,500 calories or so of intramuscular glycogen.

Protein supplies the least amount of energy and is usually omitted from consideration. If fat and carbohydrate sources are plentiful, protein supplies about 5% of energy sources. As much as 15% of energy sources may derive from protein if muscle fat and glycogen are depleted.

Figure 1-4 depicts the contribution of fat and carbohydrate to energy pro-

Figure 1-4

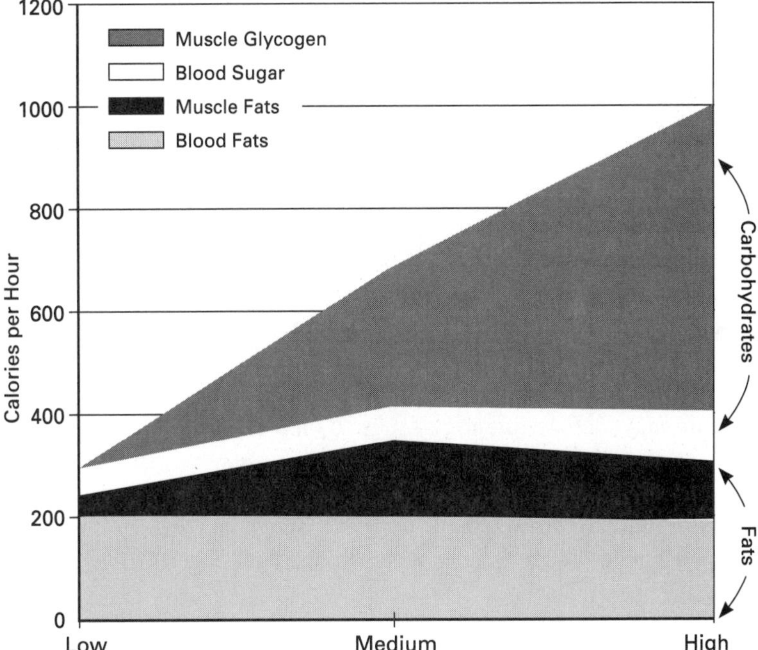

Contribution of energy sources at selected exercise intensities.

duction in a 140-pound athlete when energy stores are plentiful. Low activity corresponds approximately to a heart rate of 65% of maximum, moderate activity to a heart rate of 75% of maximum, and high activity to a heart rate of 90% of maximum.

As previously noted, traditionally the amount of carbohydrate energy used was believed to be higher than in Figure 1-4. Carbohydrate metabolism was originally calculated on the basis of respiratory exchange ratios—determined from the relative concentrations of carbon dioxide and oxygen expired. Newer techniques have suggested that fat contribution is greater than was previously determined.

The most recent studies show that at low levels of exercise intensity, about 85% of calories are supplied by fats; at medium levels, about half. At high levels of exercise intensity, 70% of energy needs are derived from carbohydrate.

At low levels of exercise intensity, most energy is supplied from fats in the bloodstream. At higher levels of exercise intensity, fat calories come from muscle stores. The absolute energy contribution from fat rises as exercise progresses from low to medium intensity, but the relative contribution declines. Intramuscular fat (triglyceride) energy at medium-intensity exercise provides less than one-third the energy of muscle glycogen. At high levels of exercise, the absolute amount of fat contribution decreases and the relative amount plummets as glycogen sources predominate.

Blood fat and blood glucose contribute to muscle energy production even at high exercise intensity levels, but the contribution is relatively small compared with that of glycogen. The contribution may increase if glucose is ingested. It is impractical to ingest fat—its utilization takes too long.

A maximum of about 250 calories per hour of ingested carbohydrates may contribute to muscle energy production. Ingesting carbohydrates spares muscle glycogen and allows exercise intensity to increase or remain high longer.

As glycogen stores are used up, exercise intensity cannot be maintained. The relative contributions of fat and protein to energy production rise. "Fat burns in the flame of carbohydrates." When glycogen is exhausted, the rate of fat metabolism also decreases. With glycogen exhaustion, muscle protein is broken down, metabolized by the liver, and returned to the muscle as blood sugar.

Training may increase the use of muscle fat and the rate of uptake of blood fat for a given exercise intensity, but at high levels of exertion, glycogen remains the fuel of choice. Without glycogen, high-intensity exercise cannot take place.

For those regularly exercising at high intensities, increasing fat in the diet is counterproductive—there is no point in sparing glycogen if the net result is that you have none to spare.

Nutrition While Riding

What We're Talking About

Nutrition during a training ride or race is one of four dietary periods for a bicycle rider. The other periods are pre-race, post-race, and non-race.

The priorities for nutrition during riding are water, calories, and electrolytes. For extremely long rides, other minerals and vitamins have some importance.

For rides under an hour, no special nutrition may be needed. For most events over an hour, concern yourself mainly with fluids and calories. For ultra-distance races over most of a day or longer, electrolytes, in addition, must be considered.

Although the order of importance is water, calories, and electrolytes, any weak link may be a performance-limiting link. It is possible, for example, for a lack of sodium to limit performance even though water and energy levels are high.

Consider an analogy. In a 40-kilometer time trial, the priorities might be fitness of the rider, bicycle-rider aerodynamics, road friction, and bicycle mechanics. This is the relative order for time spent in preparing for an event. But if your bottom bracket seizes up, all the fitness in the world won't give you a great time.

Caveats

- Individual losses and needs vary widely depending upon body size, climate conditions, acclimatization, training, and other factors.
- Recommendations for athletes occasionally differ from recommendations for health in the general population.
- Recommendations for competition do not necessarily apply to the general diets of athletes.

Nutrition Losses

FLUID LOSS

Fluid is lost primarily in the urine and through sweating. The kidneys have a tremendous ability to dilute or concentrate urine. They can rid the body of large excesses of fluids when the need arises. They can also concentrate urine if a person becomes dehydrated. Sweat rate depends upon work rate and climate (heat and humidity). During hard work in hot desert-like conditions, it is possible to lose more than a couple of liters or quarts per hour. Sweat rates have been measured up to 3.5 liters per hour and 17 liters per day.

There is a fitness and acclimatization effect in sweat production. With fitness and with acclimatization to heat and humidity, sweat is produced at lower core body temperatures—you sweat more easily. With acclimatization and training, the electrolyte concentration of sweat is decreased. Women tend to sweat less than men at the same core body temperature.

For events longer than one hour, or one-half hour in the heat, water replacement is important. Although carbohydrate or electrolyte intake may not be necessary for energy or balancing mineral losses in events under one hour, they may aid hydration by increasing the rate of water uptake by the gastrointestinal tract.

You'll notice, however, that during races, the best 40-K time trialists do not drink, even in desert events. During races at maximum effort—although dehydration worsens performance slightly—the disruption of rhythm, the time cost of drinking and the aerodynamic cost of water bottles usually justify not drinking.

MONITORING FLUID LOSS

No method is perfect, but using a bathroom scale can help determine hydration status. Although it is possible to lose or gain fat or muscle weight during multi-day events, most of the loss or gain in weight reflects hydration status. One quart of water weighs about 2 pounds. However, a scale can be misleading.

Glycogen binds, on average, three times its weight in water. Since glycogen depletion is common in multi-day events, some weight loss reflects decreased glycogen stores rather than hydration status. Glycogen stores normally average about 500 grams. No more than 2 kilograms, or 4.5 pounds of weight loss, can normally be attributed to glycogen exhaustion.

CALORIE/ENERGY LOSS

Energy loss depends upon work rate. Work rates may be up to 1,200 calories (kcal) per hour in a 40-K event.

In ultra-distance events, work rates are reduced, but duration—the number of hours of work—is increased. It is possible for a 200+ pound rider cycling 24 hours in a day to burn 15,000 calories. The typical daily energy requirement of a 150-pound racer cycling 22 hours per day is 10,000 calories. Most multi-day ultra-distance riders become calorically deficient, consuming about 85% of their daily energy expenditure.

For events longer than 2 hours, carbohydrate-in-water replacement spares glycogen and serves as a fuel when glycogen is exhausted. This helps improve performance.

High-carbohydrate diets are critical to continued high-level performance in aerobic endurance athletes who train more than three days per week. For aerobic endurance athletes, the importance of diets containing more than 65% of their calories from carbohydrates is well documented and was discussed earlier in "Diet: Why High Carbohydrates?" on page 9.

ELECTROLYTE LOSS

Electrolytes are minerals. Minerals in general are discussed in more detail in the next chapter, "Vitamins and Minerals."

Electrolyte loss is dependent upon urine and sweat loss. With electrolyte excess, significant excretion through the kidneys allows the body to normalize levels. With electrolyte deficiency, the kidneys conserve. The kidneys have the ability to vary the rate of sodium excretion, for example, by a factor of more than 100. A normal balance of electrolytes is maintained through a very wide range of intakes.

Sweat loss can result in involuntary electrolyte deficiencies after exercise lasting several hours. After hours and hours of aerobic work, the body's normal means of stabilizing electrolytes may be overwhelmed, and the body's chemistry thrown out of whack.

Electrolyte losses in sweat are listed in Table 1-4.

Table 1-4

	Sodium	Potassium	Chloride	Magnesium
Blood	140	4.0	110	1.8
Sweat	40	4.0	40	3.3

Electrolyte concentrations of blood and sweat, in milliequivalents per liter.

Sodium

Sodium is the electrolyte priority for the ultra-distance athlete. Almost everyone who is sodium depleted is also dehydrated.

For the non-athlete, the daily requirement is about 500 mg of sodium. The average Western diet contains more than ten times that amount, or more than 5 grams. Many persons consume several times this amount.

A NOTE ON NUMBERS

1,000 milligrams (mg) = 1 gram (gm)
One liter ≅ one quart
1 gram sodium ≅ 43 milliequivalents (mEq) sodium

Part of the reason this subject is confusing to many without a science background is that units of measurement vary; they may be metric units or British units. Tables with one unit of measurement often make little sense when compared with tables with other units. The symbol ≅ indicates an approximate equivalent, not an exact equivalent.

Consider sodium—an important electrolyte, or blood mineral—found most commonly in table salt. The recommended daily intake of sodium is 2,500 mg. The recommended daily intake of salt is 6,000 mg, because salt also contains chloride, which is added to the weight of the sodium.

Sodium is measured in the blood in units called milliequivalents—mEq. Typically, for example, the amount of sodium in the blood is 140 mEq. How does this relate to milligrams? There are about 43 milliequivalents of sodium per gram of sodium. Or, 1 milliequivalent is about 23 milligrams of sodium (1,000 divided by 43, since 1 gram is 1,000 milligrams).

In hot conditions one can lose a liter (quart) of fluid an hour, with 40 mEq of sodium. So that's about 1 gram of sodium—2.5 grams, or ½ teaspoon of table salt.

Table 1-5

Product	Serving Size	Sodium (mg)	Carbohydrate (gm)	Fat (gm)	Protein (gm)	Calories
Apple juice	8 oz.	15	29	0	0	116
Exceed	8 oz.	50	17	0	0	70
Gatorade	8 oz.	110	14	0	0	56
MetRx	8 oz.	195	12	1	18	130
Spizerinctum	8 oz.	133	44	2	8	233
Bananas	1 med.	0	30	0	1	125
Fig bars, no fat	2	115	23	0	1	100
PowerBar	2.25 oz.	90	45	2	10	225
Pasta sauce	4 oz.	450	7	4	2	72
Pizza	3 oz. slice	500	20	6	6	160
Pretzels	10	500	22	3	1	120
Salt, table	1 tsp.	2000	0	0	0	0
Soy sauce	1 tbs.	1300	0	0	0	0
Soup, instant	2 oz. dry	1300	44	2	7	220

Sodium and energy (caloric) content of selected foods

A chronic excess of sodium can be a factor in hypertension. The medical establishment and the popular press encourage us to reduce our average intake to about 2,500 mg of sodium daily.

There are about 40 milliequivalents per gram of sodium. So, assuming a sweat rate of 1 liter per hour, the body loses about 1 gram of sodium per hour during heavy exercise in a warm environment. After five hours of such loss, the average total daily intake of sodium may be inadequate to meet demands, and the level of sodium in the blood may drop.

For ultra-distance athletes, it is reasonable to plan on an intake of as much as 1 gram of sodium per liter of fluid loss. This is about ½ teaspoon of salt. It is preferable to eat salty foods or drinks rather than ingest salt tablets. Studies have shown that salty foods and drinks appropriately stimulate thirst, and so prevent the unintentional ingestion of dangerously high amounts of sodium.

The sodium and energy (caloric) content of selected foods is listed in Table 1-5.

Chloride

This electrolyte is usually not a big issue, because chloride most often comes along with the sodium you ingest—salt replaces both.

Potassium and Magnesium

These electrolytes are lost in sweat at about one-tenth the rate of sodium and chloride loss. Vegetables, grains, potatoes, milk, and fruit—the foods of a well-balanced diet—are common sources.

Potassium and magnesium are often packaged along with other minerals in "athletic foods"—energy drinks and bars. Although they can occasionally be a problem to replace in ultra-distance events, people who eat a diet of solid food or athletic foods are usually protected.

Bottom Line Recommendations

- For all but time trial events under one hour, drink plenty of fluids.
- It's prudent to always have carbohydrate-in-water solutions. See the chapter "Hydration."
- For multi-hour events in conditions of heat and humidity, consider consuming a salty diet or adding electrolytes to your water bottles.

Vitamins and Minerals

Vitamins

A vitamin is defined as one of a group of organic substances, present in minute amounts in natural foodstuffs, that are essential for normal metabolism. The lack of a dietary vitamin causes a deficiency disease.

Vitamins are divided into two groups: those that are soluble in water and those that are soluble in fats. The water-soluble vitamins include eight recognized B vitamins and vitamin C. The fat-soluble vitamins are vitamins A, D, E, and K.

Almost all of the water-soluble vitamins are not stored in the body and must be taken daily. Deficiency of some of the B vitamins can be observed in as little as a few days. Vitamin B_{12} is different—it is stored in the liver, sometimes for more than a year.

The four fat-soluble vitamins—A, D, E, and K—are stored in the body. It is not necessary to consume these vitamins every day. As long as your average intake is adequate, you'll be OK. Vitamins A and D may accumulate to toxic levels in the body and are associated with overdose problems.

It is difficult to diagnose vitamin deficiencies because the available tests tend to be unreliable.

Minerals

The major minerals function as electrolytes or as building blocks in structures such as bones and teeth. Electrolytes—including sodium, potassium and chloride—work as charged elements within the blood, in cells, or across cell membranes. Calcium and phosphorus function not only as electrolytes but also in the structure of bone.

In contrast to the major minerals are the trace minerals, defined as those found at a weight of less than one part per million in blood. Nine trace minerals have been identified as having a role in nutrition and have U.S. RDA or ESADDI values (see below). Five trace minerals have been considered to possibly have a role in athletic performance: chromium, copper, iron, selenium, and zinc.

Recommended Daily Allowance (RDA)

The U.S. Department of Agriculture has established guidelines for vitamin and mineral intake. Recommended daily allowances—RDAs—represent average needs, and vary depending upon age, sex, and whether women are pregnant or lactating. Some vitamins and minerals, known to be essential, have not received official recommendations for intake. Some of them have established estimated safe and adequate daily dietary intakes: ESADDIs.

The recommendations of the USDA have changed over the years. Recommended values should not be taken as gospel. Recommendations in other countries differ from the U.S. RDAs, in some cases considerably. As science continues to evolve, modifications will take place. For example, the RDA for folic acid has recently been raised to help prevent neural tube defects in the fetuses of pregnant women.

Megadoses of vitamins, defined as ten times the RDA, may function as drugs and have harmful side effects.

ATHLETES ARE TARGETED BY HEALTH BUSINESS

It is often said, "Americans have the most expensive urine in the world."

Many athletes take scores of pills daily. Vitamin and mineral supplementation is big business. Companies try to distinguish themselves from others by claiming that their formulations are superior. As you'll read below, there is very little evidence that *any* supplementation is worth it.

Food is likely to contain as yet unknown important substances. Vitamin and mineral pills may not meet our as yet unknown needs.

Mainstream scientists do not recognize any significant difference between natural and synthetic vitamins or between different formulations. The cost of such supplementation can be very large and is not worth it.

Most of us get all the vitamins and minerals we need with a good diet. If you want to be safe, you can take a multi-vitamin/multi-mineral such as Centrum daily. Centrum costs a few dollars per month at the local grocery store or pharmacy. Spend more money than that on vitamins, and you are probably wasting your money. Even worse, you may experience side effects and decreased performance.

"Fad Compounds"

Some substances called vitamins are not recognized as such by the scientific community. The promotion of these substances often benefits the seller's pocketbook more than it does the performance of the athlete who purchases them. "Vitamin B_{15}"—pangamic acid—is an example of a substance sold to athletes with no recognized status in the scientific community and little to recommend it beyond hope and a placebo effect.

Quasi-medical sources will suggest that certain herbs, spices, or other substances may be helpful. Sometimes alternative nutritional compounds contain naturally occurring drugs that do have some action. These effects are not always beneficial, and sometimes they are harmful. These compounds are often illegal for athletic use.

Some of these compounds are discussed more fully in the chapter "Ergogenic Aids" on page 34.

If you're still not convinced, think of it this way: *There is enough known nutritional information on which to concentrate your time, effort, and money. You needn't invest in the unknown.*

Decreased Performance with Vitamins and Minerals

Many athletes take out "extra insurance" and consume large doses of almost all known vitamins and minerals "just in case." One problem associated with supplementation is that an excess of one vitamin or mineral may interact with and affect the absorption or metabolism of another vitamin or mineral. Because of such an interaction, a deficiency may result even though the other vitamin or mineral is present is "normal" amounts. Balance is sometimes more important than quantity.

Many studies have shown that supplementation can *decrease* performance. Sometimes doses beyond the RDA cause side effects. Megadoses act as drugs and may cause death.

- Vitamin B_3 has been shown to prevent the release of fatty acids. This might adversely affect endurance performance. Excess B_3 can also trigger the release of histamine, causing flushing, itching, asthma, and gastrointestinal problems. Excess B_3 can cause gout, diabetes, and liver damage.

- Vitamin B_6 can cause depletion of glycogen stores. An excess can cause neurologic problems, including clumsiness and gait disturbance. It can interfere with the action of prescribed medicines.
- Folic acid excess can camouflage vitamin B_{12} deficiency, allowing neurologic problems associated with B_{12} deficiency to progress unchecked.
- Vitamin C excess can cause decreased levels of vitamin B_{12}, increase estrogen levels, and cause diarrhea and kidney stones.
- Vitamin A excess can cause headache, loss of appetite, vomiting, hair loss, itching, bone pain, and kidney and liver damage.
- Vitamin D excess can cause increased calcium in the blood and kidney stones.
- Vitamin E excess can cause malaise, gastrointestinal problems, blurred vision, headache, bleeding tendencies, and possibly hypertension.
- Vitamin K excess can interfere with the action of prescribed medicines and cause jaundice in a newborn infant.
- Calcium excess can cause kidney and neurologic disease.
- Chromium excess can cause kidney failure and lung cancer.
- Copper excess can cause liver and kidney disease, anemia, and mental deterioration.
- Fluoride excess can cause mottled teeth, gastrointestinal problems, muscle contractions, and heart disease.
- Iron excess can cause liver failure; diabetes; testicular atrophy; arthritis; and heart, skin, and neurologic disease.
- Magnesium excess can cause tremor, spasm, rapid heart rate, and high blood pressure.
- Manganese excess can cause headaches, weakness, cramps, impotence. Parkinson-like symptoms, and psychosis.
- Molybdenum excess can cause gout.
- Selenium excess can cause hair loss, fingernail abnormalities, emotional problems, and fatigue.
- Sodium excess can cause fluid retention and high blood pressure.
- Zinc excess can cause stomach ulcers, pancreatitis, lethargy, anemia, fever, nausea, and lung problems. Zinc excess reduces "good" cholesterol (HDL) and increases "bad" cholesterol (LDL). It is also associated with impaired immune function and decreased copper absorption.

Increased Performance with Vitamins & Minerals

THE CLAIMS—PURPORTED BENEFITS

All the vitamins, with the exception of vitamin K and biotin, have been claimed to improve performance. Performance enhancement has been claimed for the minerals chromium, copper, iron, selenium, and zinc. Only five of these claims have been shown in scientific investigations to have any possible merit.

POSSIBLE BENEFIT OF VITAMIN-MINERAL SUPPLEMENTS

- The antioxidant vitamins are vitamins C, E, and beta-carotene (a precursor form of vitamin A). Some scientists think that they prevent "free radical" damage—a type of damage to body cells, which might lead to cancer or heart disease. They were popular in the early nineties, but more recent evidence has found an opposite effect. The consensus is still that they are important, but the initial enthusiasm has been tempered.
- Vitamin C has been shown to improve performance in some studies but has also been shown not to improve performance in about an equal number of studies. The best-designed studies tend to show no effect. Vitamin E has not been shown to improve performance.
- Pantothenic acid was shown to result in reduced oxygen use for a given workload in one group of runners. Other studies have not found a similar effect.
- Zinc has been shown to improve some measures of muscle performance in one study. Other studies have shown no improvement with zinc.
- Iron has been shown to improve performance in athletes who were iron deficient and anemic. In the absence of anemia, it has not improved performance.

Studies have failed to demonstrate performance benefit for vitamins A, D, B_1, B_2, B_3, B_6, B_{12}, biotin, folic acid, copper, and selenium.

CONCLUSION

Get the recommended daily allowance from food. Supplement modestly. Megadoses or expensive vitamins not only may fail to improve performance but may be toxic.

Vitamin and Mineral Tables Explained

On the following pages the requirements for vitamins and minerals are listed along with their sources, benefits, functions, and other information.

REQUIREMENT

The first column shows the RDA. Quantities are given in milligrams or micrograms. Where an RDA does not exist, the Estimated Safe and Adequate Dietary Intake (ESADDI) is given if known. The figures apply to adults, aged 19 to 50. Athletes, adolescents, and pregnant or lactating women may have up to 50% increased requirements.

SOURCES

This column lists common food sources of the vitamin or mineral.

INCREASED NEEDS

Some nutrient needs are known to increase with athletic activity, caloric intake, medically prescribed drugs, diseases, alcoholism, pregnancy and lactation, or other conditions. Although RDAs may increase in women who are pregnant or lactating, there are as yet no official guidelines for athletes. If well-established increased needs are known, they will be listed in this column.

ATHLETE DEFICIENCY

Whether or not deficiency of this nutrient is common in athletes is noted in this column. Deficiency studies are subject to error. Most deficiency studies rely on the subjects' recall of their diet histories and the accuracy of current U.S.D.A. estimates of the nutritional composition of foods.

Biochemical tests to assess nutritional deficiency are more accurate. Unfortunately, few such studies have been performed. Deficiencies related to alcohol or other drugs and diseases are not reflected in the incidence of deficiency in athletes.

Weight-Controlled Athlete Deficiency

Specific athletes may be on calorie-controlled diets. Ballet dancers, gymnasts, and wrestlers commonly restrict their caloric intake in order to improve their chances in athletic competition. These athletes are the most likely to have deficient intakes. The scientific study of these athletes is specifically targeted by some researchers. When such study has been reviewed, the incidence of deficiency is noted in this column.

FUNCTION

The accepted scientific actions of the nutrient are listed in this column.

DEFICIENCY

The disease or symptoms of the deficiency disease associated with the nutrient are listed.

PURPORTED BENEFIT

There are two issues:

- Is a deficiency of the nutrient associated with impaired performance?
- Will extra, or supplemental, nutrient enhance performance? A threshold value may exist for optimal performance. It may be that a certain dose pre-

vents a deficiency state but that supplementation only up to a certain level improves performance. Whether or not actual benefit has been shown, claims of possible benefit are listed in this column.

EVIDENCE OF HARM

Some nutrients have toxic side effects, and some may worsen performance. Where such information is available, it is summarized in the table. It is also expanded upon under the heading "Decreased Performance with Vitamins and Minerals," above.

EVIDENCE OF BENEFIT

Studies may have been performed to assess performance loss that accompanies vitamin or mineral deficiency, or performance improvement with supplementation. Studies may or may not have been performed on athletes.

Performance on a bicycle is different from performance in other sports. The beneficial effects, if any, in one sport, may not be applicable to bicycling. Studies have usually been performed on college-aged men and women, so findings are not necessarily applicable to master or junior athletes.

The results of studies are noted in this column. If a study shows a positive effect, it is noted as *Yes*. If a study shows no effect, it is noted as *No*.

Table 1-6 **Vitamins and Minerals: Requirements and Sources**

Read the text "Vitamin and Mineral Tables Explained" preceding these tables.

Vitamin	Requirement*		Sources[†]	Increased Needs‡	Athlete Deficiency	
	M	F			General	Weight-Controlled
Fat Soluble						
A	1,000	800 μg	Carrots, vegetables, dairy, meat	Drugs, alcohol	Rare	10–20%
D	5–10	5–10 μg	Milk, sun, fish, eggs, butter	A, C, P&L	Rare	
E (alpha-tocopherol)	10	8 mg	Oils, wheat germ, vegetables, nuts	A, drugs, disease, P&L	Some	40–60%
K	45–80	45–65 μg	Vegetables, liver, milk			
Water-Soluble						
B_1 (thiamin)	1.2–1.5	1.0–1.1 mg	Grains, meat, legumes, nuts	A, C, alcohol, diabetes, cancer, fever, P&L	Rare	8–25%
B_2 (riboflavin)	1.4–1.8	1.2–1.3 mg	Milk, vegetables, grains, meat	A, C, alcohol, burns, trauma, drugs, P&L	Rare	
B_3 (niacin)	15–20	13–15 mg	Meats, yeast, grains, legumes	A, C, drugs, diseases, P&L	Rare	7–11%
B_6 (pyridoxine)	1.4–2.0	1.4–1.6 mg	Meat, nuts, fruit, cereals, yeast	A, alcohol, drugs, P&L	40%	
B_{12} (cobalamin)	2.0	2.0 μg	Meat, milk, eggs	A	Rare	<15%
Biotin	30–100	50–100 μg	Most everything		Rare	
Folic acid (folate)	150–200	150–400 μg	Liver, yeast, vegetables, legumes	P&L	?50%	
Pantothenic acid	4–10	4–7 mg	Grains, legumes, meat		Rare	?
C (ascorbic acid)	50–60	50–60 mg	Citrus fruit, vegetables	P&L	Rare	7–20%

Mineral					
Calcium	800–1,200	800–1,200 mg	Milk, cheese, vegetables	Drugs, disease	
Chloride	1,700–5,100	1,700–5,100 mg	Salt	Diuretics	Rare
Chromium	50–200	50–200 μg	Mushrooms, apples, nuts, asparagus	A	Some
Copper	1.5–3.0	1.5–3.0 mg	Crab, vegetables, fruit, nuts, seeds		Rare
Fluoride	1.5–4	1.5–4 mg	Meat, shellfish, legumes, grains		Rare with fluoridated water
Iodine	150	150 μg	Iodized salt, seafood		Rare
Iron	10–12	10–15 mg	Meat, fish, legumes, vegetables		Menstruating women
Magnesium	270–400	280–300 mg	Vegetables, nuts, legumes, grains	Disease, alcohol, diuretics	Rare
Manganese	2–5	2–5 mg	Meat, shellfish, vegetables, cereal		Rare
Molybdenum	75–250	75–250 μg	Root vegetables		Rare
Phosphorus	800–1,200	800–1,200 mg	Meat, milk, grains, additives		Rare
Potassium	1,875–5,625	1,875–5,625 mg	Milk, fruit, vegetables, fish	Diuretics	Rare
Selenium	40–200	45–200 μg	Root vegetables	A	
Sodium	1,100–3,300	1,100–3,300 mg	Salt, cured meat, cheese, olives		Rare
Zinc	15	12 mg	Shellfish, grains, meat, legumes	A	

* mg, milligrams; μg, micrograms.

† Sources: vegetables = dark-green-leafy vegetables; grains = whole grains and enriched flours.

‡ Increased needs found in A = athletes, C = caloric consumption, P&L = pregnancy and lactation.

Table 1-7 **Vitamins and Minerals: Effects Related to Exercise**

Read the text "Vitamin and Mineral Tables Explained" preceding these tables.

Vitamin	Functions*	Deficiency	Purported Benefit	Evidence of Harm	Evidence[†] of Benefit
Fat-Soluble					
A	Antioxidant	Night blindness, ↓appetite	Tissue repair	Yes	No
D	Bone m	Rickets, abnormal bone	Bone formation	Yes	No, Yes: 1
E (alpha-tocopherol)	Antioxidant	Nerve and muscle damage	↑tissue repair	Yes	No: 8; Yes: 3
K	Clotting	Bleeding	None		
Water-Soluble					
B_1 (thiamin)	Carbohydrate m, co-e	Beriberi, weakness, ↓endurance	↑endurance ↑performance, ↓fatigue	Non-toxic	No
B_2 (riboflavin)	Aerobic m, co-e	Burning mouth, eyes, anemia	↑aerobic performance	Non-toxic	No
B_3 (niacin)	Aerobic m, co-e	Pellagra — diarrhea, dermatitis, dementia	↑energy, ↑performance	Yes	No
B_6 (pyridoxine)	Glucose & hg p, m	Skin, seizures, anemia	↑endurance	Yes	No
B_{12} (cobalamin)	RBC production	Anemia, neurologic	↑endurance, ↑performance, ↓fatigue	Non-toxic	No
Biotin	Glycogen formation, co-e	Rare	None		No studies
Folic acid (folate)	Nucleic acid and RBC p	Anemia, fatigue, neural tube defects	↑endurance, ↑performance, ↓fatigue	Yes	No studies
Pantothenic acid	Fatty acid m, co-e	Rare	↑aerobic performance	Non-toxic	No & Yes
C (ascorbic acid)	Antioxidant, collagen	Scurvy — ↓appetite, weakness, bleeding	↑tissue repair, ↑performance, ↓colds	Yes	No & Yes

Mineral					
Calcium	Bone	Rare, bone	None	Yes	
Chloride	Electrolyte		None		
Chromium	m, potentiates insulin	Rare, diabetes	↑muscle formation, ↓fatigue	Yes	?
Copper	RBC formation, m	Anemia, bone	↑aerobic performance	Yes	No studies
Fluoride	Teeth		None	Yes	
Iodine	Thyroid		None		
Iron	O_2 transport & delivery	Fatigue, anemia	↑performance, ↓fatigue	Yes	No
Magnesium	Electrolyte		None		
Manganese	Bone & cell reproduction	Bleeding	None	Yes	
Molybdenum	m	?Cancer of esophagus	None	Yes	
Phosphorus	Electrolyte, bone		None		
Potassium	Electrolyte		None		
Selenium	Antioxidant	Rare, ?heart disease, muscle weakness	Tissue repair, ↓fatigue	Yes	No
Sodium	Electrolyte		None	Yes	
Zinc	m, tissue repair	↓appetite, dermatitis	↑anaerobic performance, ↓fatigue	Yes	Yes: 1

* Function m, metabolism; p, production; hg, hemoglobin; O_2, oxygen; co-e, co-enzyme.
† Evidence of benefit may refer to benefit beyond deficiency states. See discussion preceding tables.

Ergogenic Aids

Ergogenic aids are ingested substances that are said to improve performance. Some are banned; some are not. Some are dangerous, some safe. Being banned has nothing to do with dangerousness, only with what the governing bodies of the sport have said is banned. Although some banned substances are dangerous or have side effects, many are not. Most banned substances do not have a beneficial effect on performance. That's because very few substances, banned or not, improve performance. Legality, another topic, is a criminal issue. Some ergogenic aids require a prescription. Let me be clear: If a substance is banned, illegal, or dangerous, it cannot be recommended.

If you compete, you should assume that anything you ingest except "real food" is banned unless you know otherwise. If you need to know about a substance, call the United States Olympic Committee drug hotline at 800-233-0393.

Some over-the-counter decongestants, used for colds and the flu, are banned. Some nose sprays are banned. Many teas and herbal remedies contain banned substances. Many pain pills, high blood pressure medications, and asthma medicines are banned. Assume that any substance is banned unless you know otherwise.

If ingested substances are going to improve performance, it is usually because strength, oxygenation, or anaerobic tolerance is improved. The following is a list of the most common ergogenic aids, their properties, side effects, status (banned or not, legal or not, need for prescription), and my recommendations as to their use.

Amino Acids and Enzymes

Not banned.

Remember, amino acids are the building blocks of protein. If you consume protein in your diet, you are probably getting many times the amounts hyped in most supplements. There is little evidence that any amino acids or biochemical enzyme supplements have any value. A large U.S. nutritional retailer was fined $2.4 million by the Federal Trade Commission for promoting free-form amino acids as a stimulator of growth hormone production. Branched-chain amino acids are purported to be able to be a fuel source and also to decrease tryptophan uptake by the brain, which may reduce exercise fatigue. *Not recommended.*

Anabolic Steroids

Banned. Prescription drugs.

Good studies regarding anabolic steroids are few. They probably do help to increase muscle mass by stimulating protein synthesis. This increases muscular strength. The use of anabolic steroids requires workouts to achieve benefit. Anabolic steroids may increase hemoglobin levels, which may result in increased oxygen-carrying capabilities of blood and increased aerobic capacity.

STEROID PROBLEMS

The big medical problem with steroids is that many athletes use doses far beyond those that are safe for improved performance. These are the athletes who tend to suffer serious side effects. The side effects include aggression, fluid retention, acne, liver abnormalities, development of male sex characteristics (deeper voice, more hair, breast atrophy) in women, and shrinking testicles in men. Steroids are illegal and the risks are great if an athlete using them is caught. They can be obtained only with a prescription or on the black market.

Avoid.

Antidepressants

Not banned. Prescription drugs (e.g. Prozac, Zoloft).

A few preliminary studies show that they can help performance. There are sound physiologic reasons why they may work. The side effects include jitteriness, insomnia, and sexual dysfunction (delayed orgasm). They may be helpful in hard-training athletes. They are very helpful in depression, and since overtraining and depression are linked, they can be helpful to some athletes.

Avoid without medical need.

Anti-inflammatories—NSAIDs

Not banned (aspirin, ibuprofen, others).

Non-steroidal anti-inflammatory drugs reduce pain and inflammation. Some may have a helpful effect on blood flow. They have relatively few side effects; gastrointestinal upset is the most common.

Consider.

Bee Pollen

Not banned. No evidence of ergogenic effect.

Not recommended.

Blood Doping and Erythropoetin (EPO)

Banned. Prescription drug.

Blood doping is blood transfusion. EPO is a hormone that stimulates the body to make more red blood cells. The purpose is to boost the oxygen-carrying capacity of the blood. This probably works and is hard to detect. An increase in blood thickness is a problem. EPO has been linked to several cycling deaths and is too dangerous to use.

Avoid.

Caffeine

Banned limits.

In quantities up to the equivalent of several cups of coffee, caffeine can be very helpful for many individuals. It stimulates the central nervous system, dilates the heart arteries, stimulates the heart, and may help fat metabolism. It helps get some people going and reduces perceived exertion. *Disadvantages:* It is a diuretic (promotes dehydration) and causes gastrointestinal distress. It is currently banned in levels over 12 micrograms per milliliter of urine—equivalent to about 8 cups of coffee.

Consider.

Calories

They are vital for events lasting more than a couple of hours. Sugar solutions of up to 6% are accepted by almost all authorities. Concentrations beyond that amount may cause gastrointestinal disorders. Drinking carbohydrate and protein solutions (metabolic optimizers) during the glycogen window and supplementing calories during endurance events with MCTs—medium chain triglycerides (shorter than usual fatty acid chains) are current hot topics.

Endorsed.

Carnitine

Not banned.

Carnitine, touted as increasing fat metabolism, can be synthesized naturally in the body from the amino acids lysine and methionine. Minor evidence suggests an ergogenic effect, but several studies show no effect. Some forms of carnitine are associated with muscle weakness.

Not recommended.

Chromium

Not banned.

Lose fat? Build muscle? This mineral is essential to the function of glucose metabolism, and high-sugar diets are associated with increased urinary losses. The role of chromium in protein synthesis is the basis for claims of its anabolic benefits. Positive studies are of low quality, and current studies do not show a benefit. The long-term safety of the picolinate version is uncertain—side effects may include cancer and anemia.

Not recommended.

Corticosteroids

Some are banned.

These hormone products may be applied topically, inhaled, or injected. They can help a wide variety of inflammatory medical problems and so help performance. Inhalation of corticosteroids, or injection into a muscle or joint for local problems, requires prompt notification of the United States Olympic Committee and National Governing Body (USA Cycling).

Avoid without medical need.

Creatine

Not banned.

The body's own creatine phosphate is important for short, anaerobic efforts. The question is whether oral ingestion succeeds in getting creatine to the muscles to improve performance. Some recent preliminary evidence suggests this is possible, usually when the amount of consumed carbohydrates is also increased. Other studies have shown orally ingested creatine to worsen performance. It's of doubtful value in endurance events. Creatine is associated with water retention and cramping, and it is expensive.

Not recommended.

DHEA

Banned.

DHEA is dehydroepiandosterone: the major androgen hormone produced by the adrenal gland. Its effects result from its conversion to testosterone. This natural hormone declines with age, but its importance (relative to other androgens produced elsewhere in the body) is uncertain. Because of its anabolic action, it could help performance. Of course, all anabolics are banned. Although a drug, it is unregulated and is sold in health food stores. Dosage, formulation, and quality are uncertain, as are long-term side effects.

Avoid.

Dimethyl Sulfoxide—DMSO

Not banned.

There is little evidence of any effectiveness. DMSO does have side effects.

Avoid.

Herbs and Exotic Compounds—"Adaptogens"

Some are banned.

With herbs, it's difficult to know just exactly what you are ingesting. If they have an important pharmacological action for athletes, it's usually because they contain a known substance, perhaps banned. Guarana is caffeine. Ma huang is ephedrine, a stimulant. These substances have been found in bishop's tea, Bringham tea, chi powder, Energy Rise, Ephedra Exel, joint fir, Mexican tea, Mormon tea, popotillo tea, squaw tea, Super Charge, and Teamster's Tea.

Many herbal products have diuretic actions. Herbs with diuretic actions include horsetail, lily of the valley, saw palmetto, sarsaparilla, and uva ursi.

Many popular energy bars and products contain these banned substances. Many products with the words *Charge, Pep, Rocket, Thunder,* or *Turbo* contain these substances.

Many herbs marketed for their ergogenic properties have no known studies demonstrating any effect. This applies, for example, to ginseng.

Not recommended.

Glycerol

Not banned.

Glycerol, a three-carbon molecule, forms the backbone of triglycerides. It may also act to increase hydration, but so does a little extra salt in the diet.

Studies have had mixed results. Cramping and weight gain are side effects.

Not recommended.

Hydroxymethylbutarate—HMB

Not banned.

Purported to spare protein, HMB is a proprietary product (sold by a company with a patent). There is little evidence of any effectiveness in trained athletes.

Avoid.

Inosine

Not banned.

Inosine is a nucleic acid, and there is no evidence of an ergogenic effect. There are theoretical reasons why it may actually worsen performance.

Not recommended.

Melatonin

Not banned.

May help jet lag. A hormone produced by the pineal gland, melatonin is currently unregulated by the FDA and is sold in health food stores. Its potency is uncertain, and its short- and long-term side effects are not known.

Not recommended.

Minerals

Women with heavy periods may be deficient in iron. There is little evidence that calcium, phosphorus, sodium, chloride, potassium, magnesium, selenium or iodine are likely to be lacking in most athletes' diets. Chromium is discussed above.

Phosphate may improve performance when taken several days before competition. It may act by buffering lactic acid, increasing glycolysis, and by increasing 2,3 DPG—an enzyme that helps the blood release its oxygen to muscles. Bicarbonate may have some effect for events up to several minutes in duration by acting as a buffer for lactic acid. Both phosphate and bicarbonate may cause stomach upset and diarrhea.

Some minerals taken in excess have been shown to *worsen* performance. Read the text under "Vitamins and Minerals" starting on page 23.

Consider.

Narcotics

Some narcotics are banned. Some are prescription drugs. They work by deadening pain. Almost all narcotics worsen cycling performance because they depress the central nervous system. Codeine, dextromethorphan, lomotil, and imodium are narcotics or derivatives that are not banned.

Avoid.

Nootropics

Not banned.

Stimulants including acephen, aniracetam, centrophenozine (meclofenoxate), cleregil, euclidan, gutamine, heptamol, 3-hydroxypyridine, ionol, nicametate, oxiracetam, pantogam, phenibut, piracetam, pyritinol, sodium oxybutyrate, syndocarb (mesocarb).

There are no valid scientific studies on these compounds, even though they are in widespread use in Europe.

Not recommended.

Pentoxiphylline (Trental)

Not banned.

This prescription drug may work to increase blood flow, but there are no known studies of its effects on athletes. It is used by some to counteract the blood clotting/sludging effects of EPO.

Not recommended.

Peptide and Glycoprotein Hormones and Analogues

Banned. Prescription drugs.

HCG (human chorionic gonadotropin) can work to make the testosterone: epitestosterone ratio normal, thereby masking steroid use. ACTH (adrenocorticotropic hormone) has steroid-like effects. GH (growth hormone) has steroid-like effects. They all have potentially significant side effects.

Avoid.

Stimulants—Sympathomimetics

Some are banned. Some are prescription drugs. Some are illegal.

This class includes amphetamines, cocaine, adrenaline, and similar compounds: ephedrine, pseudoephedrine, isoetharine. Many asthma and decongestant medicines contain these substances.

Most athletes perform maximally without their use. They do not make you stronger. They may increase alertness, reduce fatigue, and increase competitiveness and hostility. They can "perk" you up, like a cup of coffee.

In low doses they are probably not especially helpful, and in high doses they are potentially dangerous, causing nervousness, anxiety, palpitations and heart irregularities, poor judgment, dependence, addiction, and death.

Most of these compounds are banned. The only asthma medicines approved in this class are inhaled albuterol and terbutaline. If you have a medical need for these compounds and have a USOC waiver for their use, they may help you, and it's okay to use them.

Avoid without medical need.

Vanadyl Sulfate

Not banned.

Vanadyl sulfate is purported to mimic the activity of insulin, but there have been no performance studies in humans.

Not recommended.

Vasodilators

Not banned. Prescription drugs.

Nitroglycerin, for example, is reportedly used by some athletes near the end of a competition, not before or during. No studies are known. There are serious side effects.

Avoid.

Vitamins

If you eat a balanced diet, the usual advice is that you don't need any extra vitamins. A general multivitamin, costing about a dime a day, may be used as insurance. Anything additional is a waste of money. Side effects from high doses do exist. Some vitamins taken in excess have been shown to *worsen* performance.

"Vitamin B_{15}"—pangamic acid—is an example of a substance sold to athletes with no recognized status in the scientific community and little to recommend it beyond hope and a placebo effect.

Read the text under "Vitamins and Minerals," starting on page 23.

Water

The most important "ergogenic" aid, not banned, perfectly legal. *Endorsed.*

Read the text under "Hydration" on page 50.

Ergogenic Quackery: Maxxta Makes You Fasta

WHAT WE'RE TALKING ABOUT

High-carbohydrate or high-fat diet? Power Bars or PR? Creatine? Antioxidants? Laetrile? Chelated vitamins and minerals? Melatonin? Yohimbe?

DHEA? Breathe-Right Nasal Strips? Echinacea? Garlic? Ma huang? Ginseng? *Siberian* ginseng?

The headline SCREAMS "Improved performance with the new wonder miracle supplement—Maxxta."

One little seed, raising the possibility of improved performance, is planted in your brain. Will it make you faster? Does the fact that the current world champion uses it mean that it really works? Does the fact that your friend uses it—and says it works—mean you should try it?

Snake oil was the magical elixir in times not long past. And regardless of the age, it seems there is no shortage of athletes or ordinary folk looking for the magic pill or potion to make them younger, go faster, be thinner, or cure the incurable. How can you know what is real and what is a sham?

BE A SKEPTIC

Perhaps the first requirement is a healthy dose of skepticism. A multitude of products have been claimed to improve performance, retard aging, or make one go faster. But in fact, very few substances have ever been shown to work at all.

The personal testimony of others may be interesting, but it's no secret that such declarations are often without merit. The profit motive is, unfortunately, frequently present. Even the most skilled observer or scientific mind is often subconsciously influenced into thinking that something is happening when the substance is actually bogus.

When I started time trialing, racing 10 miles against the clock, I read that caffeine might help. I did a dozen time trials my first year. I was positive that I went better when I got that caffeine boost from my secret potion—coffee yogurt. Only years later did I learn that the company that produced the yogurt used coffee-flavored extract and that there was no caffeine at all in my magic go-faster food!

SCIENCE IS REQUIRED

Scientific study is the way to go. The word *science* is frightening to some and makes others suspicious. But it's really quite simple: In the scientific method, a question is asked and an experiment is performed. Enough people participate for long enough to enable some conclusions to be drawn.

For example, one simply looks at what happens to two groups, one taking the "good stuff" being tested, the other taking a similar-looking or similar-tasting stuff—a placebo, without active ingredients. Because believing in something influences not only those taking the product but also those conducting the experiment, it's important that neither group knows who's getting what until the results are in, the "code" of the experiment is broken, and the results are analyzed.

SCIENCE HAS LIMITATIONS

The problem is more complicated, however. Although some fear "science," others endorse it too readily. "Science" is fallible.

Although the scientific method is the way to go, you've got to look at how the real world operates before blindly accepting scientific results.

Take ten researchers looking into whether or not Maxxta makes you faster. Suppose Maxxta is a new substance, not well studied. There are no reports yet in the scientific community about it. In fact it's doubtful whether anyone cares about it at all. Of the ten researchers, nine look at the product and find no reason to pursue their study. Early studies either show no effect or just don't seem promising enough to warrant more research.

No one, not the scientific nor the lay press, is interested in reporting that something unknown doesn't work. Only positive findings on new products make their way into the press.

But one of the researchers does see some positive effect. This researcher gets really excited. This researcher contacts a product-development company, and the stuff is marketed. The public relations people are called in. The next thing you know, *Runner's World, Bicycling, Men's Health,* and *New Woman* publish articles, and people are talking. The results look impressive.

Athletes are charged up about the whole idea. Members of the national team get wind of the research and wonder whether they should be taking Maxxta. The national coaches and physiologists wonder too, and they decide they'd better try it.

The manufacturer says fine, let me send you some product to try. The manufacturer notes in its advertising that the national team is using Maxxta. This gets everyone else thinking they'd better use it too. And since Maxxta costs a lot, you'd better believe you're getting something for your money.

A couple of years go by, and Maxxta is the rage—everybody is buying it. Some of the original ten researchers scratch their heads and remember that they found no effect. Most of them are respected Ph.D.s and M.D.s. A few review their earlier efforts and restudy whether Maxxta works. A couple of them report their negative findings at the next poster session of the American College of Sports Medicine.

Runner's World and *Bicycling* get hold of the negative studies. Now they are interested, because now that everyone thinks Maxxta works, a negative study is news. But by now four years have passed.

Maxxta doesn't really work. Nine out of the ten original researchers found no effect. The one who found a little effect and sold the product might have been an honest researcher, but honestly came up with fluky results. The magazines did their job and published the original positive information because it *was* news.

So what? Somebody made a profit. Some new product will come along to replace Maxxta.

The bottom line is that you do need good scientific research to establish whether something works. But you also need to be cautious. Understand that selection bias in reporting and publishing means what works is published, and what doesn't isn't—until it's news to say otherwise.

PROMOTING DECEPTION

Products may be mixed with other substances to market them more effectively. Energy bars, for example, apparently cannot stand on their own. The original intent of providing ready-to-eat calories won't sell enough bars unless consumers believe they should pay for the added value of vitamins and minerals.

Low cholesterol becomes a buzzword, and foods that never could have had any cholesterol are now marketed as having none. *Diet, lite, natural,* and other misleading and meaningless words are added to advertising copy to sell product.

BE CAUTIOUS WITH HEALTH FOOD STORES

You can get vitamins, minerals, and "natural" foods from the health food store. You can also get herbs and other "natural remedies."

There are many reasons to be cautious about this practice. Substances sold as remedies in health food stores are unregulated. "Natural" isn't necessarily any better than synthetic—natural mushrooms or hemlock can kill you too!

In any given bottle,

- It's uncertain what the active ingredients are.
- It's uncertain whether substances are in a form that will be available for your body to use.
- It's uncertain what else is mixed in with the pills.
- It's uncertain whether the pills are safe.
- It's uncertain whether the product is formulated consistently from batch to batch.
- It's uncertain whether the same ingredients are present in the next bottle.

A report in *Consumer's Reports* on a certain brand of ginseng showed that amounts of ginseng per dose varied by a factor of 10, even though the bottles were labeled as having the same quantity. Whether there is any good reason to believe ginseng works is another matter entirely.

Supplements have always been hot in America. They are held to a lower standard than drugs. As Brad Stone, an FDA spokesperson, notes, "A company must show a drug is safe and effective before it gets approved. With supplements, the burden of proof is after the fact. The FDA must show that a product is unsafe to take it off the market."

RECENT EXAMPLES

A few years ago, creatine was the magic pill for all athletes. Most recent published studies of it have failed to show any benefit for aerobic athletes.

Antioxidants have been the rage for several years. Recently a medical study was ended prematurely because of increased deaths from cancer in some groups taking beta-carotene.

Melatonin has been touted as a cure-all for everything from sleep disorders and jet lag to cancer and AIDS. By some accounts it can prevent or cure diabetes, cataracts, Alzheimer's disease, schizophrenia, and epilepsy. Its proponents have claimed that it can reverse the aging process and energize a lackluster libido. A recent editorial in *Nature* quotes Dr. Fred Turek, Director of the Center for Circadian Biology and Medicine at Northwestern University, Chicago: "The data are simply inconclusive." Says Dr. Richard Wurtman, director of clinical research at M.I.T., "Melatonin has been vastly overhyped."

Chromium picolinate is a supposed cholesterol reducer, muscle builder, and weight loss aid. A recent study found that this supplement caused chromosome damage in cultured cells from hamster ovaries. "Taken long-term at high doses, chromium picolinate could potentially be a human carcinogen," says Diane Stearns, Ph.D., a researcher at Dartmouth College in Hanover, New Hampshire. The FDA has received complaints on chromium, citing side effects such as heart arrhythmias, nervousness, and tremors.

OUTRIGHT QUACKERY

It is charitable to think that a researcher or journalist is after the absolute truth. Sometimes the truth is ugly. The profit motive is large in the motivations of any industry. Marketing costs may be huge. Somebody must pay for those full-page ads. Selling the product is how people make their living. While most don't deceive intentionally, some do.

The Bottom Line

You already have enough to concentrate on to help you stay fit—for example, a balanced diet and plenty of rest. And don't forget the biggest and most important ingredient of all. I use it, and people have accused me of cheating. It's called—training. *Caveat emptor.*

Ergolytics

What We're Talking About

We've learned about ergogenic aids—substances that supposedly help improve performance. A great deal is written about materials or methods that may enhance exercise capacity or otherwise augment human performance.

Now let's concentrate on the things that work to undermine your performance, sometimes without your knowing it.

There's quite a long list of ergolytics: substances that worsen performance. Most athletes don't hear enough or think enough about these substances.

The list starts with nutrition: the energy sources you eat, the vitamins and minerals. It progresses to drugs, many of them medicines you might take under a doctor's orders. And then there are a few substances that you take thinking they'll make you better, when in fact they make you worse! Don't be surprised to see some of the substances you saw listed under "Ergogenics" also listed here.

I don't mean the following listing to be comprehensive. I just want to get you thinking about what you put into your body or what you do that may worsen your performance. I'll discuss common, representative problem areas, then briefly list other ergolytics in those areas.

Nutrition

ENERGY SOURCES

Too many calories. If your total intake of calories is too high, you're going to gain weight. Extra fat may help you to float when you're swimming, but it worsens performance in most endurance aerobic events.

Wrong composition of calories. If you are an endurance aerobic athlete, performance comes from glycogen—a storage form of carbohydrate. If you use your glycogen daily, you've got to replace it, and that means a diet high in carbohydrate. Fad 40-30-30 diets (40% carbohydrates, 30% fat, 30% protein) may be popular, but without the carbohydrate fuel, you can't maintain high-energy output.

VITAMINS AND MINERALS

Sure, we all need vitamins and minerals. But too much of some of them worsen performance. An energy bar or two on a ride, plus a multi-vitamin tablet in the morning, add up to multiples of our RDAs for many of us. Although *five* vitamins and minerals have been shown to possibly benefit human performance, *nineteen* have been shown to worsen performance or cause disease when used in excess.

Nutrients of particular interest to athletes include the following:

- *Vitamin B_3* prevents the release of fatty acids. This can adversely affect endurance performance. Excess B_3 can release histamine, causing flushing, itching, asthma, and gastrointestinal problems. Vitamin B_3 can cause gout, diabetes, and liver damage.
- *Vitamin B_6* can cause depletion of glycogen stores. An excess can cause neurologic problems, including clumsiness and gait disturbance.
- *Vitamin C* excess can increase estrogen levels.
- *Copper* excess can cause liver and kidney disease, anemia, and mental deterioration.
- *Iron* excess can cause liver failure; diabetes; testicular atrophy; arthritis; and heart, skin, and neurologic disease.
- *Selenium* excess can cause fatigue.
- *Zinc* excess can cause anemia.

Other potentially ergolytic nutrients include Vitamins A, D, E, and K; folic acid; calcium; chromium; fluoride; magnesium; manganese; molybdenum; and sodium.

Only vitamins C and E, pantothenic acid, zinc, and iron have been shown to have a possibly positive role in athletes—and studies on these substances are mixed, at best. Studies have failed to demonstrate a benefit for vitamins A, D, B_1, B_2, B_3, B_6, and B_{12}; biotin; folic acid; copper; and selenium.

As you exercise more, you eat more. As long as you don't eat junk food, your intake of nutrients will rise appropriately. Stick with no more than two or three times the RDAs, and you won't get into too much trouble.

Street Drugs

ALCOHOL

In twenty years of medical practice, I hardly ever met anyone who consumed alcohol who admitted that they did not drink in moderation, even though I was taught that 10% to 25% of patients in a general family practice are alcoholics.

Beer is the number one choice of athletes. Those French studies showing a reduced risk of heart disease with a nightly drink of red wine notwithstanding, alcohol is a poison.

You might not think that drinking before riding is common, but alcohol has the dubious distinction of being the number one killer of teens and young adults in the U.S. One-third of Americans who die each year from bicycle accidents are found to be riding under the influence of alcohol.

The calories in alcohol displace other valuable food sources, and alcohol consumption is associated with many nutritional deficiencies, including deficiencies in folic acid, iron, and B vitamins. Although portrayed as a replacement beverage in advertising, it is a poor replacement fluid—possibly worsening dehydration and not providing sodium or carbohydrate for glycogen refueling. Excess alcohol may impair the liver's ability to store glycogen. Alcohol may negatively affect heart rate, stroke volume, work capacity, peak lactate levels, blood pressure, and respiratory dynamics. It is poisonous to muscle cells. It increases the risk of dehydration and hypothermia. It slows reaction times. It can worsen exercise-induced asthma.

Attention, especially guys: Alcohol is associated with decreased testosterone levels, which is associated with reduced muscle mass and decreased oxygen-carrying red blood cells.

Studies examining cycling performance time to exhaustion always show worse performance by subjects who have consumed alcohol—even low to moderate doses in Bond's 1983 study. Perception of exercise exertion did not change—the athletes thought they were doing fine. In another study, aerobic performance decreased more than 10%.

Of course, alcohol is associated with many other, non–cycling-specific problems, including behavioral/psychiatric disorders (impaired judgment, secondary depression, disturbed sleep, anxiety, personality change), withdrawal (hyperexcitability, toxic psychosis, alterations in perception, hallucinations), fetal alcohol syndrome, increase in bad cholesterol and fats, seizures, muscle disease, ulcers, and cirrhosis of the liver.

OTHER COMMON ERGOLYTIC STREET DRUGS

- *Tobacco,* including *smokeless tobacco.*
- *Marijuana.*
- *Cocaine.*

Medical Drugs

ANTIHYPERTENSIVES: DIURETICS, AND BETA-BLOCKERS

A sizable number of us take medicines for high blood pressure. Although exercise may reduce the need for these medicines in some people, high blood pressure is a big factor in heart attacks and strokes—diseases that account for almost half of all deaths. Doctors take hypertension seriously, but unfortunately, many of the drugs used for hypertension worsen high-level human performance.

Beta-blockers include Inderal (propranalol) and Tenormin (atenalol). If your blood pressure medicine ends in "alol," it's probably a beta-blocker. In one study, a cyclist riding at a steady prescribed pace without Inderal in his system became exhausted after 79 minutes. At the same pace, with 80 milligrams of Inderal in his system, it took him only 23 minutes to become exhausted. His heart rate was reduced from 163 to 129 beats per minute. A similar effect was produced by 100 milligrams of Tenormin. According to *Consumer Reports on Health,* "Beta-blockers reduce the body's ability to regulate temperature, so drink up before, during, and after workouts; exercise in the cooler hours ... and consider scaling back workouts in really hot weather."

Fortunately, most medically prescribed ergolytic drugs have substitutes that treat the medical problem without the ergolytic effect. Be sure to ask your physician whether prescribed drugs worsen performance and whether there is a substitute. For example, in the case of hypertension, an angiotensin-converting enzyme (ACE) inhibitor may be a better choice.

OTHER COMMON ERGOLYTIC MEDICAL DRUGS

- *Antacids.* The over-the-counter availability of cimetidine (Tagamet) and other so-called H_2 blockers has helped many with acid problems. But-Tagamet is also an anti-androgen—it lowers testosterone levels, and so reduces muscle mass, reduces the red blood cell count, and worsens performance.
- *Antibiotics.* Their ergolytic effects are probably overstated. I recommend taking antibiotics if a doctor feels they are needed, rather than suffering through an illness without them.
- *Antidepressants.* Some are associated with ergolytic effects.
- *Oral antifungals,* such as ketoconazole, now commonly prescribed for toenail fungus, can be ergolytic.
- *Antihistamines* can help allergies or other problems that worsen performance, but in some individuals the drugs themselves can reduce performance.
- *Eyedrops* used for glaucoma, such as timolol, are beta-blockers, which can be absorbed into the body. Studies have shown that they can worsen performance.
- *Sleeping pills.* May have a hangover effects, which worsen performance.
- *Cough suppressants,* commonly codeine or other narcotic derivatives.

So-called Ergogenics

CAFFEINE

Many studies have shown that caffeine can improve performance, but it can worsen it as well. Interrupted sleep, inadequate sleep, anxiety, and headaches are all common side effects and can worsen performance. Those dependent on caffeine are also subject to withdrawal symptoms, which may include fatigue, personality changes, and an inability to perform workouts.

ALTITUDE TRAINING (TRAINING AT ALTITUDES ABOVE SEA LEVEL)

How many elite athletes have followed their coaches' or others' wisdom to train at high altitude? Altitude adaptation can be important for upcoming events at high altitude. But training suffers; intensity cannot be maintained, and so some aspects of fitness decrease. In addition, many athletes who train away from home and are not used to it end up not training as well.

OTHER POTENTIALLY ERGOLYTIC ERGOGENICS

- *Erythropoetin (EPO).* Sure, this blood-augmenting hormone can improve human performance. But death due to thickening of the blood and blood clots will slow you down in a hurry.
- *Anti-inflammatories.* Although many athletes find that a couple tablets of aspirin or ibuprofen (Advil, Motrin) can be helpful before a ride, occasional side effects are a potential problem. A possible worsening of performance has been reported in a minority of studies.
- *Phosphate sodium.* This substance is one of the few that has been shown to improve performance in many studies. But gastrointestinal side effects, including cramping and fluid retention due to the sodium component, can worsen performance too.
- *Bicarbonate.* Lactate buffering with bicarbonate of soda has been practiced for years. But many athletes suffer cramping and diarrhea, which may make performing even a 1-minute kilometer bicycle race impossible.

Hydration

Good hydration is important in successful bicycle riding. It's easy to get dehydrated; over-hydration is rare. Replacing liquids that are lost through exercise is one of the easiest and important aids to performance in most endurance sports. A conscious effort to drink may be required—most athletes do not voluntarily drink enough.

Why Water?

Proper fluids allow the body's cells to function optimally. Maintaining good hydration is essential to maintaining your strength in riding. Blood is about 50% fluid. The reduction of blood volume from dehydration affects performance quickly.

Thirst Sensation

If you are thirsty, you are dehydrated. Your body responds to dehydration with a sense of thirst, so dehydration has already happened. Also, the older we get, the slower our body's thirst response becomes.

Look for Clear Urine

You know that your *blood* is well hydrated when your urine is clear. Two caveats: B vitamins may color the urine, and, conversely, clear urine doesn't guarantee that you are well hydrated.

Cell Dehydration

Lost blood fluid volume is quickly replaced by drinking water. Cell dehydration, however, is a different case. The cells of your body are mostly water. Fluid loss from the cells may take many more hours, or even a day or two, to replace. It is possible to experience cell dehydration, drink a lot, have clear urine, and still be modestly dehydrated in the cells.

When you drink, the fluids travel from your gastrointestinal tract into your bloodstream. The kidneys immediately sense a fullness of the blood vessels and begin to eliminate what they perceive as surplus fluid. However, your cells may not have had time to absorb fluids and so remain dehydrated.

It is a little like a plant that hasn't been watered for some time. The soil is dry, and the roots and leaves are dehydrated, so you water it. But before the plant can absorb the water, it has run through the porous, dry soil, leaving the plant still dry.

Prehydration

If you are racing in hot weather, or racing several races within a short span of time, particular attention must be given to adequate prehydration in the days before racing. You want not only your blood vessels to be hydrated but your cells to be filled as well. Consciously drink plenty of fluids, and look for clear urine for several days before racing.

How Much Should You Drink?

If you are riding in cool weather, one water bottle an hour is the standard recommendation. It may or may not be enough.

How Much Water Can You Lose?

I sometimes ride from Del Mar to San Clemente, California, and back—about 85 miles. On the way I drink from my two large water bottles. In San Clemente I buy two or three bottles of fluid. I drink one there and use the rest to refill my water bottles. On the average, I leave at 147 pounds and come back at about 142 pounds. If I'm 5 pounds lighter at the end of the ride, it means I am still down more than 2 quarts of fluid.

Once I rode a 40-K time trial in 90°+ heat and high humidity. I drank 2 gallons within an hour of the end of the ride—and I still wasn't tanked up.

I once went on a desert trip with my wife and rode a century. Both of us needed to replace almost one-third of our weight in fluids that day. I drank 45 pounds—almost 5 gallons. That's 20 quarts. That's eighty 8-ounce glasses of fluid!

It's easy for the body to use a lot of fluid quickly.

Electrolyte Additives

What is lost with sweating and hard breathing (the lungs moisturize air) is mostly plain water. Some electrolytes or salts (sodium, potassium, chloride, etc.) are lost, but it's mostly water. Water is the most important item to replace.

Expensive athletic drinks or solutions aren't necessary for usual athletic activity. The most important value of electrolytes is that they improve taste and so encourage riders to drink. If dehydration occurs, electrolytes may help the body absorb and retain water.

Aerobic endurance athletes who exercise daily for more than a couple of hours can deplete the body's reserves of electrolytes, principally sodium and chloride. Eating salty foods, or adding up to ½ teaspoon of ordinary salt to each 16-ounce water bottle, is recommended under these circumstances. See the chapter "Nutrition while Riding" for a more complete discussion.

Calorie Additives

For rides longer than about 30 miles, studies have shown that solutions containing carbohydrates allow for improved performance in comparison with plain water. A few studies have shown that calories can help performance even during shorter distances. And calories in solution help water and electrolytes to move from the gut into the bloodstream.

"Sports drinks" may provide this. Soft drinks may provide this. One-third to one-half strength fruit juice (apple, orange, etc.) may also provide the calories as well as replace some of the modest electrolyte losses that occur with sweating. Note that some individuals do not tolerate fruit sugar (fructose) as well as other sugars.

MAXIMIZING CALORIES

Add as many calories as you can to gain maximum benefit. But if you add too many—if the solution you are drinking is a concentrated one—the stomach will empty more slowly, and the gut will send in water from the body to neutralize the concentration of the fluid you have drunk, causing you to temporarily dehydrate yourself further. Your intestines may also try to eliminate this overly concentrated solution so you may get cramps or diarrhea. Studies have shown that for most people exercising at moderate levels of exertion, a 6% to 8% simple carbohydrate solution is the maximum that can be tolerated. This is represented by A in Figure 1-5.

Doubling the concentration of a glucose solution from 6% to 12% will double the calories but usually cause gastrointestinal upset. This is represented by B in the figure.

You may be able to pack more calories into a given fluid volume by combining a variety of sugars. A 6% fructose and 6% glucose solution, for example, may cause less gastrointestinal upset than an 8% solution of either of these simple sugars. Further, increased water and electrolyte movement from the gut into the bloodstream may take place, as different mechanisms of transport are involved with these two simple sugars. This is represented by C in the figure.

You may also be able to pack more digestible calories into a given fluid volume by using glucose polymers. These glucose chains increase calories without increasing the number, or concentration, of particles. This is represented by D.

Figure 1-5

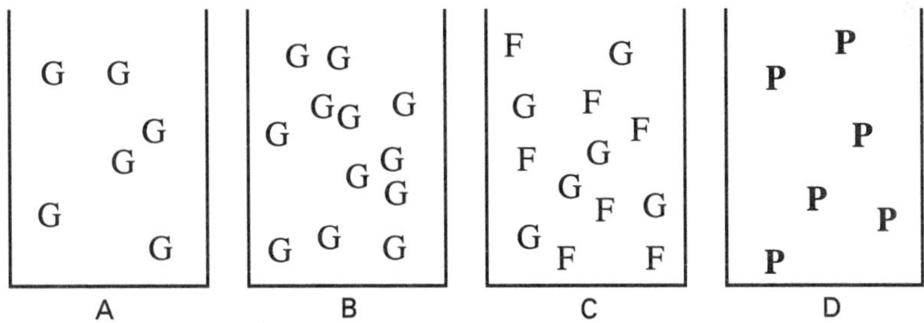

Optimizing sugar solutions. "A" represents a 6% glucose solution. "B" represents a 12% glucose solution. "C" represents a 6% glucose and 6% fructose solution. "D" represents a 6% glucose polymer solution. The text describes the diagrammed concepts.

Even if you are only going on a short ride, it makes sense to always have some calories in what you drink. They may not be necessary for performance today, but who knows—maybe you'll end up traveling farther than you thought, or perhaps it will help you keep your glycogen topped up and allow you to perform better tomorrow. The rider who trains daily or rides more than 150 miles a week is always fighting glycogen depletion.

SPORTS DRINKS

Sports drinks can be helpful. Before- and during-exercise sports drinks don't contain protein or fat. These ingredients are sometimes included in recovery drinks. Some riders cannot tolerate the fruit sugar (fructose) in fruit juices, whereas other simple carbohydrates, such as glucose, may not present a problem. As described earlier, because the intestines often react to the number of sugar particles in solution, stringing together single-molecule sugars into chains of glucose polymers or maltodextrins may allow for more calories to be consumed without increasing gastrointestinal upset.

There is some evidence that adding a small amount of protein to drinks may improve recovery. This is the basis for the addition of modest amounts of protein to some athletic drinks designed to be consumed after riding.

MAKE YOUR OWN SPORTS DRINK

1 cup unsweetened fruit juice
¾ teaspoon salt
¾ cup sugar
2 ¼ quarts water

Makes 2½ quarts—five 16-ounce water bottles, each with about 150 calories.

Real Juice

We were back at my car after a 60-mile ride. I had a gallon thermos of drink in the trunk. A previous Olympian was with me. He was thirsty. I gave him some purplish fluid.

"What's that?" he said, swallowing eagerly. "That's great. Is it Cytomax, or a new energy drink?"

"Not too strong?" I asked.

"No. Terrific. Is this why you go so fast?"

"Don't know, but it helps," I said.

"What is it? Who makes it?" he asked again.

"It's from the grocery store," I said. "Tropical Fruit, made by Dole. 100% pure juice, diluted about 50/50 with water."

"Wow!" he said. "Real juice!"

Caffeine Additives

For occasional use, to get you going 20 minutes before a ride, caffeine in solution (coffee, tea, Coke or Pepsi, etc.) can be useful. It can also be useful for time trials or about an hour before the end of a long ride to get you through to the end.

Caffeine is a stimulant, and I do not recommend it for regular use. It can cause bowel cramps and diarrhea. Caffeine is also a diuretic, which means it will also act to dehydrate you. Use it at your own risk, and remember that the race will continue without you if you have to find the bushes.

Alcohol?

Alcohol during a ride is rotten. Like caffeine, it is a diuretic, robbing you of fluid. It forces you to urinate and it slows you down. It makes your legs heavier. Physical activity increases the intoxicating effect of alcohol. With your judgment impaired, you can easily crash.

Alcohol has minimal, if any, nutritive value beyond calories. It is associated with impaired physical health as well as decreased performance. Alcohol is associated with many vitamin deficiencies.

A few studies show a small benefit to some aspects of health of roughly 1 ounce daily. These studies are overwhelmed by the innumerable studies demonstrating the toxic effects of alcohol to health, performance, and society.

Make It Taste Good

Plain warm water doesn't taste great. A little flavor, a little sugar, a little electrolyte makes it taste better. Cool water goes down more easily. Having good-tasting fluids allows you to drink more.

Water Is Best

Remember, *hydration* is from the Greek for *water,* and that's what you chiefly need.

Tips to Help You Lose Weight

If you want to lose fat, you've got to create a caloric deficit. Since glycogen binds about three times its weight in water, and since glycogen is often lost when dieting begins, initial rapid weight loss may be due to loss of glycogen and water, not fat. It's reasonable to lose a pound or two a week. More than that may be too rapid, leading to loss of muscle mass and other problems.

One pound of fat equals about 3,500 calories. The only way to lose a pound a week is to have an energy output that is 500 calories higher than energy intake, on average, for the seven days of the week. This 500-calorie energy difference can come from increased energy needs (an increased activity level) or a decreased caloric intake (dieting).

Changes you incorporate into your daily regimen should be gradual and sustainable. You are presumably looking to modify or change behavior patterns for the long term.

It is possible to lose too much weight. Read the text under "Too Thin?" on page 269 in the "Women's Health" chapter.

Activity

If you increase your activity and eat the same amount of food, you will lose weight. Daily exercise not only helps you lose weight but relieves stress. It may promote increased coordination, body tone, cardiovascular fitness, and social interactions.

Find an activity that you enjoy. Exercising when you don't like what you are doing is a chore, one you are not likely to continue. An exercise group, club, or team may provide extra motivation to keep you active.

Dieting

1. Eat only when you are hungry.
2. Buy a calorie counter. Set your calorie goals. Learn the nutritional value of foods.
3. Buy no-fat or low-fat foods. Avoid purchasing foods that get a high percentage of their calories from fat.
4. Arrange to do all your eating in only one place. For example, eat only in the kitchen or only in the dining room.
5. Avoid eating while you are doing something else. It is easy to eat when you don't really need or want to, for example, while watching TV or at a ball game.

6. Avoid having tempting foods around with lots of calories. If you open the refrigerator and a piece of cake is staring you in the face, it is hard to avoid eating it. Keep "no-no" foods out of sight, stored away in cupboards.
7. Snacks should be available that are low in calories and satisfy a desire to have something in your mouth. Keep carrots or celery sticks in the refrigerator as snack foods.
8. Do not have second servings readily available. At dinner, for example, do not bring the pot to the table. Make it an effort to get that second helping. Keep the food on the stove. If you are in the dining room and you have to get up and go all the way to the kitchen to get the pot, chances are you won't have that second helping. If the pot is on the table, it is easy to put "just a little more" on your plate.
9. Serve smaller portions. Serve portions attractively, but on smaller plates. Restaurants do this all the time. Large plates are served, then a smaller soup bowl is placed on the plate, and then inside the soup bowl an attractive small portion appears. Your brain sees the large plate and thinks you are getting a lot. But there really is not that much there!
10. Eat slowly, and chew each piece more thoroughly. Sometimes people eat so fast that their brain does not have time to catch up with their stomach. They shovel the food into the stomach before the brain realizes it's there, and find that they have eaten more than they need to be satisfied.
11. Shop with a list. Don't shop for food when you are hungry. Studies show that shopping without a list on an empty stomach is the best way to buy junk food you don't need or want.
12. You only lose fat by starving. Let's agree that starvation is unpleasant. Eat a normal breakfast and lunch, but eat a light supper and you lose fat while sleeping—like a hibernating bear. This is more agreeable than starving while conscious.
13. When you are hungry, don't focus on your hunger. Think instead how much healthier you'll be. If you want to climb better, visualize yourself climbing faster. See yourself keeping up with your friends, or passing your buddies.
14. Keep a diet diary. Notice when you eat. Be a detective; figure out why. It is not unusual for people to skip breakfast and have a light lunch in order to eat fewer calories. Then they pig out at supper. Or, they starve during the day, then wake up at midnight, go to the refrigerator, and pig out. A light supper meal might prevent overeating when hunger strikes later.
15. Consider enlisting support from friends and relatives, or from a support group: Weight Watchers, TOPS (Take Off Pounds Sensibly), or weight classes offered through other sources.

Not Recommended

- *Crash diets, fads, diet pills* (they contain caffeine, decongestants, or amphetamines). You may lose weight initially, but if you don't change your basic eating and exercise habits, they are only a temporary fix. Some medical evidence suggests that up-and-down weight gain and loss—yo-yo patterns—may be harmful. It is better to lose weight slowly and continuously.
- *Skipping meals.* Often this leaves you so hungry that you binge later.
- *Laxatives.* These can give you diarrhea and prevent the food from being metabolized by the body. They stop working when you stop taking them.
- *Diuretics.* These get rid of water, not fat. You see immediate results from a quick loss of a few pounds, but your weight comes back the next time you drink to quench your thirst.
- *Body wraps.* "Special weight-reducing clothes" make you sweat when you put them on. They are ineffective in the same way diuretics are.
- *Magic Wands.* Actually, magic wands do work. I have been looking for one for years. Let me know if you find one.

Disordered Eating

What We're Talking About

Eating disorders include anorexia (severe food restriction with the perception that one is fat) and bulimia (overeating and ridding oneself of food by vomiting). These problems usually require professional care.

Many exercise enthusiasts and elite cyclists exhibit less severe patterns of disordered eating, including a vicious cycle of dieting, exercising, bingeing, and exercising more. Both men and women may have disordered eating patterns, although the number of women and the consequences for women may be greater. Read the text under "Too Thin?" on page 269 in the "Women's Health" chapter.

Warning signs or behaviors include the following:

- *Food restriction.* Skipping meals. Voluntary starvation. If you are thin, and perceive yourself as fat, then anorexia may be the diagnosis.
- *Talking about food or weight.* If weight is usually the subject of conversation, disordered eating patterns may be present.

- *Awareness of what others are eating.* Sure, it's okay to ask others at a restaurant if they are enjoying their meal. But if you are mentally calculating their caloric intake, you may have a problem.
- *Not eating in public.* Those with disordered eating don't want others to see or calculate what they are eating.
- *Baggy clothes.* To hide perceived obesity.
- *Feeling cold.* With food restriction, the metabolic rate slows. With the resulting decreased thyroid levels, people feel cold because their body temperature is lower.

Nutrition Tips for Cyclists

The basics of nutrition have now been outlined. A new study here, a theory there, and a little bit of commercial interest results in much misinformation or fact today that may be fiction tomorrow.

Glycogen Window

The "glycogen window" refers to the concept that a post-exercise window of opportunity exists when ingested carbohydrates can be converted to muscle glycogen more readily than at a later time. Replacing a few hundred calories of carbohydrates as soon as possible after your ride may reload glycogen to a greater extent than if you travel home, shower, and then sit down to a feed. A modest amount of protein also taken during the "window" may help glycogen rebuilding in muscle. Even better: If you can eat while you ride, even though you may not need calories for today's ride, you may improve your ability to ride with intensity again tomorrow.

Energy Bars

Energy bars are a convenient way to carry about 200 calories. But many have the texture of cardboard, and they cost a lot more than bananas, nonfat yogurt, bagels, or fig bars. Candy bars have lots of sugar, taste great, and are much cheaper. It's true that they have more fat, but on the other hand, at least one maker of energy bars believes that increasing fat content has a beneficial effect on athletic performance.

Guarana

In a word, caffeine. Guarana is a dried paste of the crushed seeds of *Paullinia cupana,* a vine cultivated extensively in Brazil. Sounds exotic—it's about as exotic as Brazilian coffee beans. Its active ingredient is guaranine, another name for caffeine.

Would you buy an energy bar that contained caffeine? Maybe, maybe not. But at least you'd see the label and know what you were getting.

This is an important objection to many "natural substances" advertised and added to energy bars or other "foods." Such substances are unregulated, and consumers often eat them without being aware of what they are ingesting. Many people who avoid caffeine because of a sensitivity to it, because they are taking other medications that might adversely interact with it, or for other reasons are unknowingly consuming such substances. Further, without knowing it, many athletes consume "prohibited substances"—legal substances, but banned for competition by various governing bodies.

Beware!

Ma Huang

This ingredient, found in some therapeutic and energizing foods and teas, almost got Alexis Grewal banned from the 1984 Olympics, which would have been a pity for him, since he managed to win the road race.

Beware of exotic-natural-ancient-alternative-homeopathic-health foods. If they do have a pharmacological action, it's probably because they contain some substance known to you in a more conventional form.

Ma huang is indeed an energizing substance—but it's also banned from competition. It has been associated with thousands of emergency room visits in the U.S., because it causes serious side effects to the heart and nervous system and can result in death. You can buy it anywhere without its exotic name—it's ephedrine, sold in the U.S. under the trade name Primatene.

Carbohydrate Gels

Relatively new, gel carbohydrate packs for energy replacement supply a convenient form of calories. The label of a typical 100-calorie packet tells you to consume 12 ounces of fluid with it. If you started out with diluted apple juice in your bottle, you'd get the same calories with less expense.

Best Fuel for Cyclists—Complex Carbohydrates, Maybe

Complex carbohydrates, such as those in pasta, breads, and grains, are thought to be the best fuel for cyclists, although many have raced successfully on a diet of doughnuts, ice cream, or hot dogs.

Of course, only a few years ago a good breakfast consisted of eggs and bacon. I'm not disagreeing with concepts of modern training, but as my wife has said, the vast majority of riders have never noticed a difference one way or the other. When we're touring, we indulge in milk shakes, ice cream, candy bars, and burgers, and we feel great.

Hector Monsalve won the points race at U.S. Masters Track Nationals a few years back. I watched Hector have a burger for dinner. Not realizing that he was racing, I was floored when 5 minutes later he slipped off his jacket, slipped on some bike shorts, and, without any warmup, won his race. It was astounding.

Many Tour de France riders still have meat for breakfast. And after years of energy bars without any fat, the tide may be swinging in favor of bars with some fat.

Modern training theory is just that—theory, or the best information we have now. In the future it will be old 1990s theory.

Protein or Amino Acid Supplements—Not

No controlled scientific study has ever shown that specific supplemental amino acids improve performance. Supplements typically provide up to 500 milligrams of amino acids per pill. An ounce of chicken provides more than 8,000 milligrams as well as other nutrients.

Although protein supplementation is popular with weight lifters and is often touted as important, no study has ever shown that more than 2 grams of protein for every kilogram (2.2 pounds) of weight has any benefit. The usual dietary recommendation is one-half of that. Excess protein not only is expensive but may be harmful.

Fat Alert

Read the labels. Just because a food sounds healthy, it isn't necessarily so. Granola, for example, can be high in fat. Muffins are popular—they taste great. Let's face it—fat tastes good—but so can bagels, which have hardly any calories from fat at all!

Low Fat Hints

- Choose low-fat cooking methods: bake, broil, poach, steam, or roast.
- Cut the margarine, oil, butter, shortening, gravies, or salad dressing you use by a third.

- Reserve high-fat foods such as chips, rich desserts, or deep-fried items as once-in-a-while choices—no more than two or three times a week.
- Pick canned or packaged foods with the least fat. Look for no more than 3.3 grams of fat per 100 calories, meaning that no more than 30% of the calories comes from fat.
- Eat trimmed lean cuts of red meat, skinless poultry, or fish. A serving size is about the size of a deck of cards.

Avoid Fatty Milk

Let's face it. If you are used to whole milk, fat-free milk tastes like water—yecch. But whole milk has fully one-half of its calories from fat. Fat-free milk has zero calories from fat, and it's a great source of protein, carbohydrates, vitamins, and minerals, including calcium. It's one of the best foods there is.

Adapt to fat-free milk as you do with any other training program. Let your body adjust. Get used to fat-free milk by drinking 2% reduced-fat milk for awhile, then 1%. Finally, choose fat-free milk.

At Home, on the Road—Don't Add Fats to Great Foods

It's easy to cheat when you are trying to be good.

- Salads are great—they have lots of vitamins and minerals and are low in fat. But scoop on a few ounces of oily dressing, and now you have lots of fat and almost no carbohydrates.
- Pancakes or waffles may be a reasonable breakfast menu item when you're on the road and can't eat your usual muesli or low-fat cereal at home. But lather on the butter or margarine that's usually provided, and fat percentage skyrockets.
- The bagel was a great choice. But gobs of butter or cream cheese ruin your good selection. Use just a dab if you must, or some jam instead.
- Use mustard instead of mayonnaise on that sandwich.
- Use plain yogurt or salsa on your baked potato instead of butter and sour cream.
- Eating a burger? Have a smaller one with mustard and ketchup, not the ½-pound burger with cheese, bacon, or mayonnaise.
- Mexican food? Choose the burrito instead of the deep-fried chimichanga.
- Almost all restaurants have lower-fat items. Often they are noted on the menu or in brochures. If not, perhaps broiled chicken that you skin yourself, a baked potato, and a salad would be a good choice.

Fruit and Vegetable Hints

- Drink juice in the morning.
- Choose a salad every day.
- Eat a hot vegetable at dinner.
- Snack on vegetables or fruit.
- Have fruit for dessert.

Fiber Hints

- Have whole-grain cereal for breakfast.
- Ask for toast or sandwiches with whole-grain bread.
- Pick whole-grain rolls or crackers.
- Eat beans at least every other day.

How Many Calories Do I Use When Riding?

Calories consumed per hour depend upon your weight, your speed, and whether or not you are climbing.

You use roughly three times as many calories per hour as the watts you produce. If you have access to a bicycle power meter, either on an ergometer or with new technology such as SRM, you can get an estimate of your power output at different heart rates.

In an article in *Bicycling* magazine, calories consumed per hour were said to be $(0.046 \times V \times W) + (0.066 \times V^3)$, where V = velocity in miles per hour, and W = weight of rider and bike in pounds. Twenty-two additional calories were said to be used per 100 feet of elevation gain for a 176-pound rider and bike. By this formula, a 110-pound woman, riding a 20-pound bike and traveling at 12 miles per hour, would consume about 190 calories per hour. A 150-pound man, riding a 20-pound bike and time trialing at 25 miles per hour, would use about 1,200 calories per hour. These figures are quite approximate. With the same expenditure of energy, aerodynamics and bicycle mechanical efficiency can make a difference of several miles an hour in bicycle speed.

Systemic Candidiasis and Craving for Sweets

According to a popular theory in the 1980s, craving for sweets was said to be due to systemic candidiasis, a yeast overgrowth. There is no scientific proof that this is true. Your energy level may be low because your blood sugar level is low, you're overtrained, or you're depressed. But candidiasis is not the reason.

Calcium Supplements

Extra calcium may help prevent osteoporosis in women, but it has no known effect on performance. Extra dietary supplementation may find its way into bones, but it doesn't raise blood levels.

Nutrition Quackery

The Food and Nutrition Science Alliance (FANSA) represents members of the American Dietetic Association, American Institute of Nutrition, American Society for Clinical Nutrition, and Institute of Food Technologists.

FANSA's Ten Red Flags of Junk Science:

1. Recommendations that promise a quick fix.
2. Dire warnings of danger from a single product or regimen.
3. Claims that sound too good to be true.
4. Simplistic conclusions drawn from a complex study.
5. Recommendations based on a single study.
6. Dramatic statements that are refuted by reputable scientific organizations.
7. Lists of "good" and "bad" foods.
8. Recommendations made to help sell a product.
9. Recommendations based on studies published without review.
10. Recommendations from studies that ignore differences among individuals or groups.

Nutrition Quiz

1. T F Protein is useful before athletic events. That's why you often hear about athletes having a steak breakfast.

2. T F Everyone needs vitamins. Athletes need so many to perform well that all athletes should take supplemental vitamin pills.
3. T F Protein is important in building muscle. Athletes wanting to increase their strength need protein shakes or supplements.
4. T F Since the body's energy system runs on sugars, soft drinks and candy bars are ideal foods.
5. T F Since being light is so important in getting up hills, it helps to be a little dehydrated before hilly road races.
6. T F Athletic drinks are required during almost all races for their nutritional superiority over plain water.
7. T F Wine or beer with your meal helps digestion.
8. T F If you are training for a long race, it helps to train without drinking. This helps to adapt your body for the effects of dehydration you can expect in the long race.
9. T F No harm comes from taking too many vitamins. It is better to be safe than sorry and take lots of supplements.
10. T F During heavy hot-weather exercise, don't forget to take extra sodium or salt tablets!
11. T F Athletes making claims for foods or vitamins usually do so because they believe in the product rather than for financial gain from endorsement.
12. T F If you eat right ("to keep fit") you won't get cancer or heart disease.
13. T F Vegetarians don't get enough protein or iron.
14. T F You should eat extra food at bedtime because your body digests it better when at rest while sleeping.
15. T F Raw unpasteurized milk is a "perfect food." Certainly it is preferred to watery fat-free milk.
16. T F Your mother was wrong. Colored green and yellow vegetables really aren't important. It's a myth that you need them.
17. T F Your mother was right. You should finish everything on your dinner plate.
18. T F Since it is primarily fats that are burned on long rides, fatty foods consumed during rides actually help performance.
19. T F When you are thirsty during a hot race, it is actually better to drink warm fluids—they are already closer to body temperature.
20. T F Diet pills or prescription diet medicines from a doctor should be used to lose weight.

Bonus A Girl Scout cookie has 7 grams of carbohydrates and 3 grams of fat. What percentage of its calories comes from fat?

Quiz Answers

Probably a lot more is not known about nutrition than is known. This area is subject to much mythology. All of the twenty T F questions are false or mostly false. The Girl Scout cookie in question has 3 grams of fat, for 27 calories, and 7 grams of carbohydrate, for 28 calories. Of a total 55 calories, 27 calories, or 49% come from fat.

NUTRITION PRINCIPLES

- Eat a variety of whole, unprocessed foods in moderation.
- Eat at least half a dozen servings of fruits and vegetables daily.
- Control your weight.
- Limit or avoid alcohol.
- Eat a diet relatively high in fiber.
- Eat fewer simple sugars—candy, table sugar, "sweets."
- Avoid junk food.
- Avoid high-fat and high-cholesterol foods.
- Avoid salty foods.
- Rely on food, not pills.
- Consider a multi-vitamin/multi-mineral supplement.

There are no absolute rules. Very different diets consumed by different people may have equal nutritional value and result in good nutrition. Occasional dietary indiscretions aren't important.

Part Two

PHYSIOLOGY

Our bodies respond predictably to exercise. Understanding how activity affects our bodies allows us to tailor our activity to produce desired outcomes. Exercise physiology, as it relates specifically to cycling, is discussed in this section.

Genetic Ability

One often hears about gifted athletes, athletes with great genes, athletes who are born. How much athletic success derives from genetic ability? How much comes from perseverance and hard work?

Are Athletes Born, Not Made? An Example: Fast Twitch Versus Slow Twitch

We're often told that racers endowed with more fast-twitch than slow-twitch muscle fibers are likely to succeed in sprinting events, and that slow-twitch fibers are more conducive to endurance riding.

This may be true in theory, but I don't recommend muscle biopsies because I think they are more likely to worry and limit riders than they are to reassure and motivate them. Who can really predict what can be accomplished?

One of the best women sprinters this country has ever produced turned out to have more slow-twitch than fast-twitch muscle fibers. If she had undergone muscle biopsy before her career took off, rather than after numerous international and world championship victories, and taken her biopsy result to heart, perhaps she would never have excelled.

Genetics? How Do You Know?

I'm not saying that genetics doesn't play a role in athletic ability or success. After all, even without training, it's evident that some people are naturals at certain sports. But how do you evaluate the sum total of genetic limitations for cycling?

Maybe you think, "My parents are such couch potatoes—do I have any hope?" Perhaps given different times or circumstances and encouragement, they would have been athletic. You just don't know. You also see some athletic parents whose kids are not interested in sports at all—they don't care about their genes because their parents have tried to push them into a sport so much they've come to hate the idea of it.

In my view, "genetics" is too often used as an excuse by a rider for why he or she doesn't excel. For that reason alone, I'd rather not place an artificial ceiling on performance by invoking genetics.

Recovery

What We're Talking About

You've gone for a long hard ride or race, and you'd like to ride again tomorrow. Or you need to ride again, because you're in the middle of a tour or stage race.

Sometimes athletes debate the merits of volume versus intensity. But it's really the *volume of intensity* that makes athletes fitter.

What do you do to help assure maximal recovery and your ability to perform the next day? How do you help prepare your body to work hard again and again?

Causes of Fatigue

Knowing the causes of fatigue helps us develop the right strategy for recovery. Fatigue has several main causes:

1. Energy store depletion
2. Metabolic—fluid, electrolyte, and other chemical depletion
3. Muscle fatigue
4. Neurohormonal

ENERGY STORE DEPLETION

The body burns energy to power your activities. The high-energy fuel of choice is glycogen, a form of storage carbohydrate found in your muscles. Replacing glycogen is crucial for repeated high-end performance, day after day.

METABOLIC: FLUID AND ELECTROLYTES

Acute and chronic dehydration limits performance. It's important to replace lost fluids. Repeated prolonged aerobic work, especially in hot and humid environments, results in sodium and other electrolyte depletion, which limits recovery and performance.

MUSCLE FATIGUE AND SORENESS

Independent of energy supply, muscle fatigue and soreness can limit your ability to perform repeated work. We know that muscle factors and energy supply are different situations, since just a few short unaccustomed weight-lifting exercises can cause muscle fatigue and soreness for many days even though glycogen has hardly been used.

NEUROHORMONAL FATIGUE

Neurohormonal fatigue is an important, though less well understood, cause of fatigue. When you're "burned out" you may be unable to work hard, yet your glycogen levels may be high and muscle soreness nonexistent. Unless your nerve cells are talking to each other and to your muscles, and unless your body's hormones are working, you will not be able to work to peak levels of performance.

Adequate sleep and rest are integral to neurohormonal fitness. (As a physician who has spent many wakeful nights taking care of patients, I can tell you that my muscles are useless at performing high-intensity exercise after a few sleep-deprived nights.)

Minimizing the Need for Recovery

Hard work demands recovery. You can minimize the need for recovery by working out intelligently. Your approach before, during, and immediately after your workout may diminish your need for recovery.

- *Warm up.* Races that start off with a bang may require as much as 1 hour of warmup.
- *Replace fluids, fuels and, perhaps, electrolytes* before, during and after your workout.
- *Cool down* after hard races or training sessions with a short recovery ride.

Fluid Replacement

One is almost always dehydrated after a hard workout. Your pre-ride and post-ride body weight can provide a clue to how dehydrated you are. A quart of water weighs about 2 pounds. If your post-ride weight is down 5 pounds, you're down a little over a couple of quarts of water.

It's important to replace lost water. Although plain water is needed for fluid replacement, fuel and electrolytes are also required. Combine nutritional needs with a sports recovery drink or a careful selection of fluids and solids. The body's glycogen is combined with water, at a ratio of about three parts water to each part glycogen. Some of your decreased body weight will be due to glycogen-water losses.

Rehydrating may return the blood volume to normal, but your weight may still be down. Your weight will not return to normal until glycogen-water stores have been replaced.

Fuel Replenishment

You need to replace energy stores quickly and efficiently after you ride. A high-carbohydrate snack of at least 200 calories within the first half hour after a ride helps get energy back into that glycogen tank. At least another 200 calories each hour for the next several hours continues to top off the tank. Current research suggests that modest protein along with carbohydrate helps this refueling process work better.

Metabolic Restoration

ELECTROLYTE REPLACEMENT

For riders riding in hot weather, losses of electrolytes, chiefly sodium, can contribute to fatigue. You'll need about ½ teaspoon of salt for every quart of water you lose. Most riders lose about 1 quart an hour in hot weather, although greater losses are possible. The average person receives 2 to 3 teaspoons of salt in the daily diet. So if your ride has lasted just a couple of hours, you're probably OK. Otherwise, it may be a good idea to eat salty snacks and food.

VITAMINS, MINERALS

For racing day after day, a standard multi-vitamin, multi-mineral pill may be a wise investment.

SECRET STUFF

Ginseng? Herbs? Adaptogens? There's a lot of lore and not much science. A new potion appears every year. With more research and time, it's possible that substances may be found to aid recovery. For the moment, be skeptical and don't waste too much money on them.

Muscle

What helps muscle recover? Does massage or stretching help? Most riders and coaches believe they do. A sauna or hot tub may be relaxing, but prolonged exposure to these methods of muscle relaxation may contribute to further dehydration and salt loss.

Neurohormonal

It's easy to understand that sightseeing, business meetings, or late-night partying could contribute to additional stress on a bicycling tour, when you could be resting—napping in bed or quietly reading, minimizing stimulation—if your goal is continued performance the next day. It's clear that rest, including sleep, is an important part of neurohormonal recovery.

The nervous system and the chemicals that are used to transmit messages between nerve cells and from nerve cells to muscle fibers are an important part of exercise activity and recovery. The dysfunction of neurohormonal factors is probably the most important cause of overtraining syndrome. Neurohormonal factors are incompletely understood and hard to measure. That doesn't mean these factors should be ignored.

Active Recovery Versus Resting

Resting—not engaging in physical or mental activity—is the usual basis of recovery. But different systems respond differently. Many trainers and physiologists believe that active recovery—for example, light training—promotes faster overall recovery. This appears to be true for high-volume riders. It is uncertain why active recovery may be more helpful than resting. One possibility is that light exercise increases the blood flow to exercising muscle and thereby speeds the repair of microscopic muscle fiber damage.

Common Errors

GETTING TO A RACE TOO EARLY

It's stressful to wait around doing nothing. It's common for inexperienced racers to arrive too early, not eat, stand around in the sun, and thereby weaken themselves before they even start.

NOT PACKING A COOLER

You've got to have fluids and fuels, not only on the bike but in your car on your way to the race start and again at the finish. Cool fluids go down more easily. Knowledge of what you should do isn't good enough if you haven't planned to take advantage of that knowledge. You'll typically want to pack at least a gallon of carbo fluids, a couple of sandwiches, a few pieces of fruit, and some energy bars, fig bars, or cookies.

HANGING AROUND TOO LONG AFTER RIDING

Standing around, chewing the fat with buddies or family after the race is pleasantly social. You've got that adrenaline high from racing. It doesn't seem to take a toll. But you're weakening yourself. You're staying out too long in the sun. You're standing on those legs instead of getting them up and resting. You're probably not eating or drinking as well as you might be back home or in your hotel room. You should be getting off your legs, cleaning up, restoring hydration and fuel, or going for a recovery ride.

NOT PLANNING FOR RECOVERY

Some riders get so used to working out that they don't go easy, relax, and let their bodies recover. The harder you work, the more you need to plan recovery days so that you can continue to work hard when it counts.

Baby Yourself

Ask any parent what babies do. "Sleep, eat, and poop." That's it. If you're racing or training day after day, that's probably one of the best prescriptions for recovery!

Training Pearl—Train Inefficiently, Race Efficiently

Since different systems have different recovery needs, by training different systems at different times it is possible to allow for recovery or partial recovery of one system while training another system.

For example, you could ride a climb as fast as possible three days a week, with rest days between efforts. Or you could climb five days a week. You could climb in a big gear two days, climb in a small gear two days, and race up one day in a moderate, efficient gear.

The big-gear climbing would concentrate on strength. It would fatigue the muscles. High-level aerobic work would not be performed. Small-gear climbing at speed would work aerobic systems without taxing the muscles. Neither big-gear nor small-gear climbing would result in speeds as high as those obtained during efficient climbing in a moderate gear.

Five-days-a-week training would result in more gains in fitness for many riders because of the increased volume and quality of work done on the different energy systems. After several weeks, the climbing race-day speed would be greater than if the athlete had continued the unvarying training program of three-days-a-week efficient climbing.

Heart Rate Training

Heart-rate monitors allow you to observe your heart rate while working out. This has revolutionized modern approaches to training.

How Monitors Are Used

- Monitors are used in designing and implementing training and racing programs because they ensure that you work according to plan. A monitor helps make sure that you work hard enough. It also helps make sure that you don't work too hard!
- Monitors help you analyze how you feel and what happens in training and in races. For some riders, monitors don't necessarily change training, but they do allow an understanding of what is going on.
- Monitors help motivation. The feedback they provide is interesting and engaging for many riders.

Maximum Heart Rate

Determining maximum heart rate (HR) is the first step in developing a heart-rate training program. For most riders, heart-rate zones for aerobic, threshold, and anaerobic work are based on their maximum HR. Many coaches and athletes attempt to determine maximum HR a few times a year in order to set training intensities.

Maximum heart rate is the highest heart rate you can achieve. For most riders, the maximum HR is the highest *accurate* number they ever see on their monitor. I say accurate because sometimes electrical wires, radio transmitters, or other sources of false readings mess things up.

INDIVIDUALIZE YOUR NUMBERS

Conventional wisdom has it that your maximum HR, in beats per minute, is 220 minus your age, but this statistical average for the population is useless for the individual. It's like saying the average person is 5 feet 9 inches tall, so all bikes should measure 55 centimeters. You need to customize your numbers for yourself, then you can get started in training efficiently.

Session maximum heart rate is the highest heart rate during a particular exercise session. Few exercise sessions attempt to achieve a maximum, so the session maximum HR is rarely near an individual's true maximum.

MAXIMUM HR CHANGES

Maximum HR is not a static or fixed number. It is simplistic to say it is genetically determined. People who are unfit may not be able to achieve their genetic potential because of a lack of muscular strength or energy to work hard. Their maximum HR will increase as they become fitter.

Once fitness has been achieved, the maximum HR doesn't change much, but it does change. Elite athletes may actually have a lower maximum HR during their competitive seasons. And maximum HR is sport- and climate-specific. More on this follows.

DETERMINING YOUR MAXIMUM HEART RATE

To obtain a maximum HR value, you need to be

1. Rested
2. Well warmed up
3. Motivated to make a maximum effort

There are any number of different ways to find your maximum HR. Here is one way:

- Warm up for at least 5 to 10 minutes. After working at a moderate pace for 3 minutes, increase your effort by about 10% every minute. This means either increasing your cadence by five to ten revolutions per minute or increasing your gearing by one gear of difficulty every couple of minutes.
- When you get to the point where it is extremely difficult to continue at pace, sprint absolutely as hard as you can for 30 seconds. Watch your heart monitor. This value should be close to your maximum.

EFFECTS OF MUSCLE MASS, EXERCISE TYPE, AND POSITION

Some riders have had their maximum heart rate determined in other sports such as running or rowing, but cardiovascular demand is proportional to muscle mass. In other words, running uses more muscle mass than cycling or swimming and hence places higher cardiovascular demands on the athlete. Body position also affects cardiovascular demand. A horizontal position presents less demand than a vertical position.

For these reasons, your maximum heart rate is likely to be different for different sports. Your heart-rate training zones are likely to be different for swimming, running, and cycling. They may even be different for time trialing or climbing.

Resting Heart Rate

Resting heart rate is determined by counting or monitoring your heart rate while you are not engaged in physical activity. It is usually measured the first thing in the morning while you are lying still in bed. Conventional wisdom states that resting heart rate is a measure of fitness and recovery. As you get fitter, your resting heart rate falls. When you are not recovered, your resting heart rate rises. Use resting heart rate as a tool in evaluation, but don't get spooked by high values. Some riders have their best performances on days when their resting heart rates are high.

FACTORS AFFECTING RESTING HEART RATE

Dehydration, fever or other illness, drugs, stress, or the environment can raise resting heart rate. For many riders, the discomfort of a full bladder, the physical activity of getting up to urinate, or the jarring of an alarm clock will raise the heart rate. Resting quietly in bed for several minutes after urinating or turning the alarm clock off will give a more accurate reading.

The value measured while one is lying flat on the back is often slightly lower than that measured while one is lying on the side.

OTHER RESTING HEART RATES

Although the morning resting heart rate is used by most people, many believe that the resting heart rate recorded after a quiet rest in bed for 5 minutes upon retiring in the evening is just as predictive of recovery.

The lowest heart rates occur during sleep. These values are obtained with a recording heart-rate monitor.

Still other athletes monitor standing resting heart rates. When you stand, your blood pressure falls. Sensors in the neck initially overcompensate for this decrease in blood pressure by sending signals that raise your heart rate. As the blood pressure returns to normal the heart rate slows, but it remains at a level higher than the lying-down resting heart rate.

Some athletes monitor these changes in heart rate, believing them to be more sensitive indicators of recovery. There are different techniques for evaluating these changes. One method is to observe the difference between lying-down resting heart rate and the heart rate 1 minute after standing. This is called *delta pulse.* Another method is to observe the difference between heart rate upon standing and heart rate 30 seconds later.

Training may lower your resting heart rate. Even so, resting heart rate is, in part, genetically determined. Many racers whom I routinely beat are surprised that my resting heart rate is as high as 60.

Time Trial Threshold

Here's a number that does matter: In a one-hour time trial, what percentage of your maximum heart rate can you maintain?

Conventional wisdom says that an athlete's time-trial threshold is 85% of maximum HR. This is too conservative. The time trial threshold of fit athletes is closer to 92% of maximum HR. The threshold as 92% of maximum heart rate for fit athletes is relevant to events lasting about one hour. In bicycling, this corresponds most closely to a 40-K time trial. For events longer than this, the threshold one can sustain will be lower. For shorter events, the threshold will be higher. As extreme examples, Race Across America (RAAM) riders often race at 60% of their maximum heart rate after the first couple of days of this ultra-distance event. Track sprinters may hold their maximum heart rate for their 200-meter sprint.

These percentages apply to well-rested, fit athletes; at moderate temperatures; at sea level. Lack of conditioning, fatigue, cold temperatures, and racing at high altitude will all lower the threshold.

Thresholds Are Differently Defined

The concept of anaerobic threshold training had its current popular bicycling origins with Professor F. Conconi's coaching of Francesco Moser for his hour records: 50.808 kilometers on January 19, 1984, and 51.181 kilometers a few days later, January 23. Sport scientists and physiologists define *threshold* differently. The anaerobic threshold is not the same as the time-trial threshold. See the chapter "Thresholds" on page 85.

Recovery Heart Rate

Here's another monitoring number that matters. After a hard effort—for example, a 10-minute time trial—how long does it take for your heart rate to recover to below 100 beats per minute? The fitter you are, the faster your heart rate recovers.

Heart Rate Economy

As you become fitter you will be able to accomplish the same work at lower heart rates. You must consider your training in terms of percentages of your own heart rate, not averages.

Table 2-1 **Heart Rate Training Zones**

Level	% Max HR	Type of Effort
Noodling	< 65	Recovery, easy
Aerobic	66–85	Club rides, warm-ups
Threshold	86–92	Time trials
Anaerobic — Long	93–96	Intervals, jumps
—Short	97–100	Sprints

Noodling

Noodling is riding under 65% of your maximum HR. Easy riding. If your maximum is about 180 beats per minute, your noodling rate is under 120 beats per minute. This is recovery riding.

Aerobic Training

Working between 66% and 85% of your maximum HR. You are training *aerobically.* Aerobic means "with oxygen." This aerobic work will improve your ability to use oxygen efficiently.

Heart-rate economy will improve. As you become fitter you will be able to accomplish the same work at lower heart rates. In other words, you will be able to accomplish more work at the same heart rate.

Recovery heart rate will improve. The fitter you are, the faster your heart rate will recover from hard efforts.

Threshold Training

This is working between 86% and 92% of your maximum HR. You are at the border between aerobic and anaerobic work. This level of work is sustainable for efforts lasting up to an hour. This is the level at which you time-trial.

Threshold level will rise. New racers commonly sustain 86% of maximum HR. As fitness improves, levels closer to 92% of maximum heart rate can be maintained.

Anaerobic Training and Racing

In this range, your heart rate may be 93% or more of your maximum HR and can't be sustained for very long. This is very hard work. You get to these levels during intervals, jumps, and sprints—red-line efforts. This is not the stuff most commuters, weekend riders, and century riders need to concern themselves with.

Training in this range is, however, vital for racers. Bicycling is an anaerobic sport—breakaways and the dropping of riders only happen when at least some racers are anaerobic or maxed out.

Efforts of this intensity preceded by periods of recovery may not result in heart rates over 93% of maximum HR. You must already be riding at high aerobic levels for these anaerobic efforts to result in very high heart rates. Remember that all efforts at heart rates above 93% of maximum HR are anaerobic, but not all anaerobic efforts result in this high a heart rate.

Table 2-2 **Training Heart Rate Guidelines**

Max HR Beats per Minute	Aerobic 66 – 85%	Threshold 86 – 92%	Anaerobic 93+%
205	135–174	175–189	190+
200	132–170	171–184	185+
195	129–166	167–179	180+
190	125–162	163–175	176+
185	122–157	158–170	171+
180	119–153	154–166	167+
175	116–149	150–161	162+
170	112–145	146–156	157+
165	109–140	141–152	153+
160	106–136	137–147	148+
155	103–132	133–143	144+
150	99–128	129–138	139+

Training Time Needed to Progress

The notion of training 20 minutes three times a week, at heart rates between 70% and 85% of maximum, is for beginners.

Competitive club riders need to train at 80% to 85% of maximum for at least 30 minutes, three times a week. It would probably be best to ride at 80% to 85% of maximum HR for at least an hour once a week or more.

Competitive racers also need anaerobic threshold work—85% to 92% of maximum HR—during these periods. This may not necessarily be a training ride; it may be race day. Of course, racing *is* training.

Factors Affecting Heart Rate

Many individual and environmental factors affect heart rate. Interpreting heart rate in the context of these factors provides better insight into its meaning.

TEMPERATURE AND HUMIDITY

Heat and humidity present increased demands on the body. To help cool the body, blood is shunted to the skin. This results in elevated heart rates.

Heart rates may be one beat higher for every 2 or 3 degrees above 70°F. Although submaximal and maximal heart rates are higher, power output—with the exception of very short maximal sprint power—is reduced.

Some riders will observe higher thresholds when training, time trialing, or racing during conditions of heat and humidity. Others will be so enervated that they are not able to perform or achieve their normal heart rates.

As in hot and humid conditions, cold weather also reduces power output and results in lower heart rates.

ALTITUDE

Threshold and maximum HR are reduced about one beat for every 1,000 feet of elevation for athletes who have trained at sea level. For a given submaximal power output, heart rate is higher.

DEHYDRATION

Dehydration places increased demands upon the cardiovascular system. For any given power output, heart rates increase.

FITNESS

As non-elite athletes become fitter, they improve their cardiovascular function and increase their sport-specific muscle mass, thereby enabling themselves to achieve higher maximal heart rates. As athletes become fitter they are able to produce more power for a given heart rate, or produce the same power with a lower heart rate.

As elite and professional athletes become fitter they become more economical. In lay terms, their bodies are more efficient. Their muscle mass remains the same or slightly decreases. Their muscles work with less cardiovascular demand, and maximum HR may actually decrease during the racing season.

MEDICATIONS AND DRUGS

Drugs may decrease or increase the heart rate. For example, beta-blockers—commonly prescribed for hypertension, migraine, and heart disease—lower the threshold and maximal heart rates.

Adrenergic stimulants, found in decongestants and asthma medications, raise the heart rate. They can also cause heart irregularities, resulting in heart rates that can be misread by heart-rate monitors.

ILLNESS OR DISEASE

Medical conditions can decrease or increase heart rate. For example low thyroid function can decrease resting, threshold, and maximum HR. Conversely, hyperthyroidism can raise the heart rate. Anemia will raise the resting and threshold heart rates, and less work will be possible at threshold.

Lactic Acid

Most of us have heard about lactic acid, a product of anaerobic metabolism. Understanding some simple facts about lactic acid helps us understand training approaches and dispels some myths about this popular buzz word.

What Is Lactic Acid?

Lactic acid is a product of metabolism. Oxygen is the catalyst that allows you to burn food to produce energy when you work. There is a limit to how much oxygen you can use: your VO_2 max. As you work at increasing workloads your body uses up stored energy. It is building up a debt that must later be repaid. A waste product of this work is lactic acid. The quantities of lactic acid produced increase dramatically during anaerobic metabolism.

Lactic acid is poisonous to your cells. It is toxic. You can tolerate only a certain amount. It's what gives "the burn." Beyond that level, the discomfort will be too great, forcing you to back off.

When lactic acid enters the bloodstream it is converted to lactate.

Why Is Lactic Acid Bad?

Lactic acid is a factor that prevents you from working harder. It decreases coordination and increases the risk of injury. According to some theories, frequent training at high lactic acid levels reduces the body's ability to produce creatine phosphate for short sprints and interferes with aerobic fitness.

How Is Lactate Measured?

Lactate is usually measured by chemical analyzers from blood samples. In sophisticated labs, lactic acid levels in muscle itself can be measured, but this method is rarely used.

What Are Typical Lactate Values?

Blood lactate is measured in millimoles per liter—mm/L. It's not important that you understand exactly what these units mean; understanding the relative values of blood lactate is.

Table 2-3 **Training Intensity and Typical Blood Lactate Levels**

Training Intensity	Blood Lactate Level (mm/L)
Noodling — recovery riding	Below 2
Endurance riding	1.5 – 2.5
Aerobic training	2.5 – 4
Threshold training	4 – 10
Intervals up to several minutes	<14
Sprints up to one minute	<20

Normally your blood has between 0.5 and 1.5 mm/L of lactate. Skilled time trialists can ride at a level between 4 and 10 mm/L of blood lactate for about one hour. Longer events are ridden at lower lactate levels. Shorter events can be ridden at higher levels.

Relationship Between Lactate and Heart Rate

A relationship exists between blood lactate values and heart rate. As workload increases, both lactate and heart rate rise. As athletes become fitter they are able to perform more work at lower lactate and heart-rate levels. The exact relationship between work, lactate, and heart rate also depends on the type of effort. For example, time trialing is associated with moderate lactate levels and high heart rates, whereas weight lifting is associated with high lactate levels and moderate heart rates.

Lactate Clearance and Lactate Tolerance

Here are two important training concepts concerning lactate: (1) Training improves the ability of the body to metabolize (or clear) lactate from the blood. (2) Training improves the ability of the body to tolerate high levels of lactic acid in the muscles.

Consider this analogy. You have a bathtub. When you turn the faucet on full blast, the tub overflows after a few minutes. You want to be able to turn the faucet to maximum and not have the tub overflow. You have two options: increase the size of the drain or increase the size of the tub. Training does both.

Why Know About Lactate Levels?

By understanding what's going on, you can be smart in your training. You can structure your training to accomplish the following:

- Improve your ability to spare carbohydrates as an energy source at submaximal workloads
- Increase the number of blood vessels, the strength of your heart, and the uptake of oxygen by your muscle cells
- Tolerate higher lactic acid levels

For more information about training, see "Selected References," on page 303.

What Effects Can I Expect from Training?

Training effects will allow you to:

- Increase the fractional percentage of the maximal heart rate or VO_2 max that you can maintain
- Ride at a higher percentage of your maximum pulse rate for the same blood lactate level
- Allow the body to metabolize lactate more quickly
- Raise the level of lactic acid you can tolerate so you can work harder
- Ride the same pace or workload at a lower lactate level

Lactic Acid May Not Be the Problem

Lactic acid is not always the limiting factor in exertion. You are not always limited by your aerobic power. Sometimes you lack muscular strength, leg speed, endurance, or motivation.

Riders often complain that their legs are heavy because of lactic acid. After anaerobic efforts this may be true, but not all muscular fatigue is due to lactic acid. Lactic acid is cleared from the muscles within 30 minutes; fatigue or soreness that lasts longer is not due to lactic acid but arises from other factors. For more information about muscle fatigue, see page 104. For more information on muscle soreness, see page 108.

Thresholds

We often hear the term *anaerobic threshold.* Occasionally we also hear the terms *lactate threshold, ventilation breaking point, ventilation threshold, heart rate breaking point, heart rate deflection point,* and *heart rate threshold.* These terms are commonly misused, causing confusion. By understanding thresholds, you'll be able to more clearly understand training theory and methods.

What We're Talking About

The energy systems used in sport are the aerobic and anaerobic systems. Metabolic or physiologic chemical pathways used by the body to produce energy can operate in the presence of, or without, oxygen.

As efforts become progressively more intense the contribution of the anaerobic pathways increases. "Pure" anaerobic efforts cannot be sustained for more than a minute.

As exercise intensity increases, several observable physiologic events occur:

- Lactic acid in muscle and lactate levels in blood increase.
- Ventilation, or breathing rate, increases.
- Heart rate increases.

These physiologic signs are used as markers for anaerobic activity, but they do not mean the same thing.

Why We're Interested

- The threshold at which aerobic metabolism is no longer sufficient for energy production serves as a marker in assessing the development of the aerobic system.

- Threshold may be used to measure the response of the aerobic system to training.
- Threshold may be used to help predict performance in aerobic sports.
- Threshold may be used in the exercise prescription to help define intensity of effort in training.

Lactate Threshold

As exercise intensity increases beyond the ability of the aerobic system to meet demand, anaerobic metabolism contributes to energy production. A byproduct of this anaerobic metabolism is lactic acid. At rest, most athletes have blood lactate levels between 1.0 and 1.5 millimoles per liter. As exercise intensity increases, lactic acid levels rise. Lactic acid levels first rise in the muscles. After lactic acid levels increase in the muscle, they "spill over" within a few minutes to increase lactate levels in the blood.

The body is initially able to metabolize the increasing lactate level in the blood to maintain a steady state, so, at first, increased workloads are associated with little or no increase in lactate levels. Then, lactate levels begin to rise in relatively linear proportion to workloads. Finally, lactate levels begin to rise exponentially with workloads.

LACTATE THRESHOLD DEFINED

Lactate threshold is the point at which blood lactate begins to accumulate rapidly with increased exercise. Here are four interpretations of this definition:

- The point at which blood lactate levels begin to rise linearly with workloads. This corresponds to about 2 millimoles of lactate.
- The point at which blood lactate levels begin to rise nonlinearly (exponentially), i.e., relatively faster than the workloads that produce them. The threshold in this definition corresponds to about 4 millimoles of lactate.
- The point at which blood lactate levels continue to rise despite no change in exercise intensity. Typical lactate threshold values according to this definition are 2.5 to 5 millimoles per liter.
- Some people arbitrarily assign the value of 4 millimoles per liter as the onset of blood lactate accumulation.

PRACTICALITIES OF LACTATE THRESHOLD MEASUREMENT

Many estimate lactate threshold from a progressive test in which intensity is increased each minute. Other test protocols increase the intensity at different intervals up to several minutes. Those who define lactate threshold as the point at which lactate levels continue to rise, despite no change in exercise intensity, perform exercise tests at much longer intervals to determine this point.

This is the current method used by USA Cycling:

- A lactate threshold is estimated by use of a progressive sub-maximal test. Then, exercise is performed for 15 minutes at three levels: slightly below this level, at this level, and slightly above this level.
- Blood is analyzed for lactate every five minutes. The threshold is defined as the highest intensity level at which the last (third) lactate level of the fifteen-minute interval remains unchanged. If this occurs at the level above the estimated threshold value, another fifteen-minute interval of verification is needed at a higher level.

"Immediate" blood lactate analyzers are needed to determine whether additional intensity levels are required in the same session.

Ventilation Breaking Point

At low levels of exercise, as intensity increases, pulmonary ventilation, or the amount of air breathed, increases in a linear manner.

As levels of oxygen uptake reach approximately 40% to 60% of maximum, ventilation begins to increase more sharply. This is often observed at blood lactate levels of about 2 millimoles per liter.

A second, sharper breaking point in ventilation and blood lactate can often be detected at oxygen uptakes equivalent to 65% to 90% of maximum and blood lactate concentrations of 4 millimoles per liter.

As lactate begins to accumulate, it is buffered by blood bicarbonate. This buffering reaction results in the formation of carbon dioxide, which increases ventilation. Some have explained that the ventilation breaking point results when blood lactate levels rise non-linearly. Curiously, however, people who lack the gene that allows blood lactate to be produced still have a ventilation threshold. So it seems that the definition of ventilation breaking point is flawed or incomplete.

Heart Rate Threshold

As exercise intensity increases, heart rate rises linearly. At some point the rising heart rate "breaks" and fails to keep pace with increasing intensity. This point is defined as the athlete's heart rate threshold. This test is of value because portable heart rate monitors are now readily available and relatively inexpensive, allowing interested riders to determine their threshold themselves. Unfortunately, many authors, physiologists, and coaches find that no discrete "breaking" point is apparent when heart rate is plotted against exercise intensity.

Figure 2-1

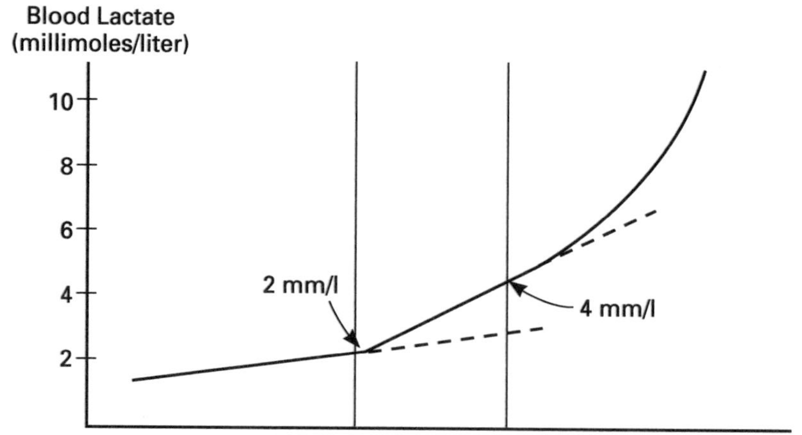

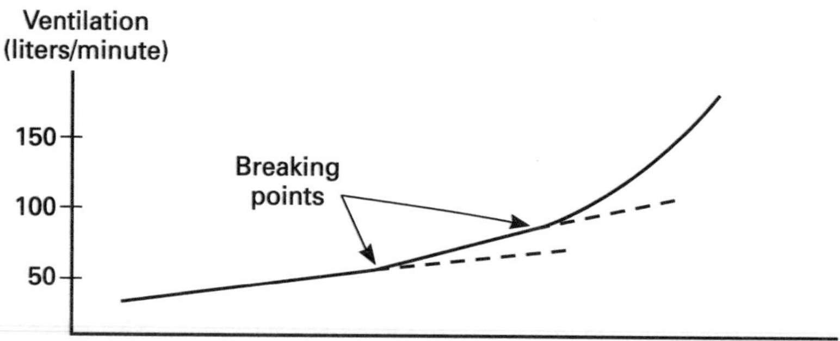

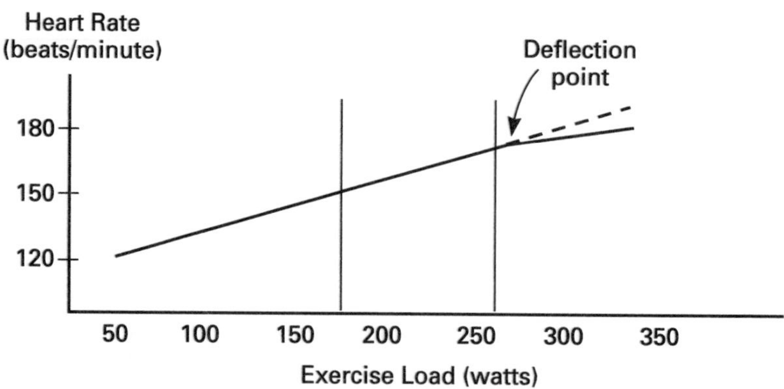

Blood lactate, ventilation, and heart rate thresholds

Anaerobic Threshold

Because some believe that the increasing blood lactate levels at the ventilation breaking point are caused by anaerobic conditions, the ventilation breaking point has sometimes been called the anaerobic threshold. But since the mechanism of the ventilation and blood lactate breaking points is incompletely understood, and it is not certain what is being measured, many avoid the term *anaerobic threshold.*

Time-Trial Threshold, Maximum Lactate Steady State

There is a popular conception that the anaerobic threshold is determined, reached, or defined when an athlete time trials at maximum pace. But clearly the intensity level at which an athlete can time trial depends upon the duration of the event. The blood lactate levels during a track pursuit of 4 kilometers are higher than those of a road time trial of 40 kilometers. For each of these events, sustainable blood lactate levels are greater than those noted by observing physiologic breakpoints. Elite riders can ride beyond their physiologic breakpoints for more than one hour.

The level of effort an athlete can sustain for a steady-state event is best referred to as the *time-trial threshold* for that event. The time-trial threshold for events of about 20 minutes is sometimes called *maximum lactate steady state.* This is what most riders really mean when they talk about anaerobic threshold, though they misuse the term in the strict physiologic sense.

Those who define lactate threshold as the point where blood lactate levels continue to rise, despite no change in exercise intensity, may interpret blood lactate threshold as time-trial threshold.

Elite athletes can time trial at 92% of their maximum heart rates for one hour at sea level and 70°F. Conventional wisdom has it that elite athletes can time trial at a level 4 millimoles of blood lactate for one hour. This conventional wisdom is wrong. Numerous investigators have found that the true figure for maximum lactate steady state is higher at 6 to 10 millimoles of blood lactate.

Practicalities and Significance

Thresholds are indicators of aerobic endurance performance and training progress. They are less suitable for predicting maximal oxygen uptake or VO_2 max. Maximal oxygen uptake is a poor predictor of athletic performance as long as the level is high for all—which is often the case in elite athletes. Power at threshold is a more important predictor of aerobic endurance performance than VO_2 max.

Blood lactate levels can be measured in the field, under training and racing conditions. This makes them a more popular marker than ventilation thresholds among coaches and investigators. Although thresholds provide a way of assessing submaximal aerobic capacity, exercise prescription remains a question of coaching philosophy. Although some coaches base training zones on thresholds, others believe that such systems are misguided.

Training Intensity

The methods of determining and measuring training intensity have evolved since the advent of heart rate monitors. Whether or not training has changed, depending upon coaching philosophy, is another issue.

What We're Talking About

How hard riders train. Measuring the effort of training.

The Conventional Method—Perceived Exertion

Before heart rate monitors, training intensity was measured in terms of perceived effort. Several scales of perceived exertion are still in use today. Endurance or "aerobic" training was either long-slow or long-steady distance. Time trial efforts, intervals, and sprints were usually performed at the maximum speed possible to complete the effort.

PROS

- Descriptive, intuitive.

CONS

- Uncertain reliability and validity.
- Easy to work too hard or too little.

Modern Training Intensity—Heart Rate Zones

Heart rate monitors have allowed training intensity to be quantified in terms of heart rate. This method allows athletes to measure their workout intensity against a standard, rather than having to guesstimate how hard they are working. My definitions and those used by USA Cycling are shown in Tables 2-4 and 2-5.

Table 2-4 **Arnie's Heart Rate Ranges**

Effort	% Max HR*	Description
Noodling	<65	Recovery riding
Aerobic	66–85	Club rides
Threshold	86–92	Time trials
Anaerobic	93–97	Jumps, intervals
	97+	Sprints

* % Max HR, percentage of maximum heart rate.

Table 2-5 **USA Cycling Training Zones**

	% Max HR*	Description
Zone 1	<65	Recovery, easy riding
Zone 2	65–72	Aerobic training
Zone 3	73–80	Anaerobic threshold training
Zone 4	84–90	Lactic acid training
Zone 5	91–100	ATP-CP training†

* % Max HR, percentage of maximum heart rate.
† ATP-CP: Adenosine triphosphate-creatine phosphate.

PROS

- Quantifiable, i.e., you can accurately measure the intensity of your workout.

CONS

- Moderately expensive. Requires heart rate monitor. Charting percent time in each zone requires a more expensive heart rate monitor and/or a computer with interface.
- Easy to neglect strength or leg speed work, which may have an intensity that doesn't correlate well with heart rate monitoring alone. Riders may focus on heart rate rather than on what they need to be doing.
- Heart rates may not rise quickly enough to reflect effort intensity during short efforts, especially with significant recovery between efforts. In sprints,

heart rates may continue to rise for a few seconds after the effort is over and may not reach near-maximal levels.

Multidimensional Heart Rate Training

When cadence or speed are specified along with heart rate, a more specific exercise prescription can be defined. For example, riding at 75% of maximum heart rate and a cadence of 50 r.p.m. emphasizes strength. Riding at 75% of maximum heart rate and a cadence of 125 r.p.m. emphasizes leg speed.

The Future—Power and Lactate

Other measurements of exercise intensity include power output and blood lactate. Riders are becoming increasingly familiar with power output in watts and blood lactate levels in millimoles per liter. Power measuring devices have been in use for several years. They remain very expensive, but their price is expected to fall in a few years. Blood lactate levels can be monitored with moderately expensive field-measurement devices similar to a blood glucose monitor. They require a finger prick to obtain a drop of blood. Just as glucose monitors have revolutionized control of diabetes, blood lactate measurement may revolutionize training intensity.

A possible future intensity table might look like Table 2-6.

Table 2-6 **Possible Future Intensity Table**

	Power	Blood Lactate
Effort	**% Threshold**	**mm/L**
Noodling	<50	1
Aerobic	75	2.5–4
Threshold	100	3.5–10
Intervals	150	6–12
Sprints	250	10–16

PROS

- May be closer to quantifying what is important in training.

CONS

- Expensive.
- Riders may focus on numbers rather than on training tasks and needs.

Science Isn't Everything

Modern physiologic measuring methods allow us to "know" what's going on. These measuring methods will be refined and improved, but always remember that they can't replace a good coaching program or a positive exercise philosophy.

VO_2 Max

We often hear about this test as a measure of athletic ability. What does it mean? How is it determined? How should you use it? What values can be expected?

What Is a VO_2 Max Test?

This test is a measure of aerobic capacity. It is a measure of how much oxygen the body can use over a given period of time. These days, it is considered the single most important test in endurance performance evaluation and prediction. A high aerobic capacity is necessary, but not sufficient, for success by elite cyclists.

Many people erroneously equate oxygen capacity with lung performance. The lungs are the first link in the aerobic chain. But the heart and blood vessels must get oxygenated blood to the muscles, and the muscles must extract that oxygen from the blood and chemically use it to produce energy. In the absence of lung disease, maximum oxygen uptake has more to do with the heart, blood vessels, and muscles than it does with the lungs.

The test measures the volume of oxygen used per minute, divided by weight. The test result is reported as mL/kg/min. This means milliliters of oxygen per kilogram per minute: the volume of oxygen (in milliliters or thousandths of a liter), per unit of weight (the kilogram), per unit of time (the minute).

The amount of oxygen two different people can use per minute may be the same, but their VO_2 max will differ if they are of different weights. If two subjects have the same absolute volume of oxygen used, the lighter subject will have the higher VO_2 max.

How Is VO_2 Max Measured?

The test is performed while the subject is exercising—usually running on a treadmill or pedaling a stationary bicycle. The athlete is required to perform more and work each minute, until exhaustion is reached. Maximum oxygen uptake usually occurs near maximum heart rates. VO_2 max tests performed during running are often 5% to 10% higher than those performed during cycling because more muscles are used in running.

- The volume of air that the subject breathes each minute is measured.
- Exhaled air is analyzed for the percentage of oxygen and carbon dioxide.
- From these values, the volume of oxygen the athlete uses each minute can be calculated.
- The athlete's weight in kilograms is divided into this value to obtain the VO_2 max.

Figure 2-2

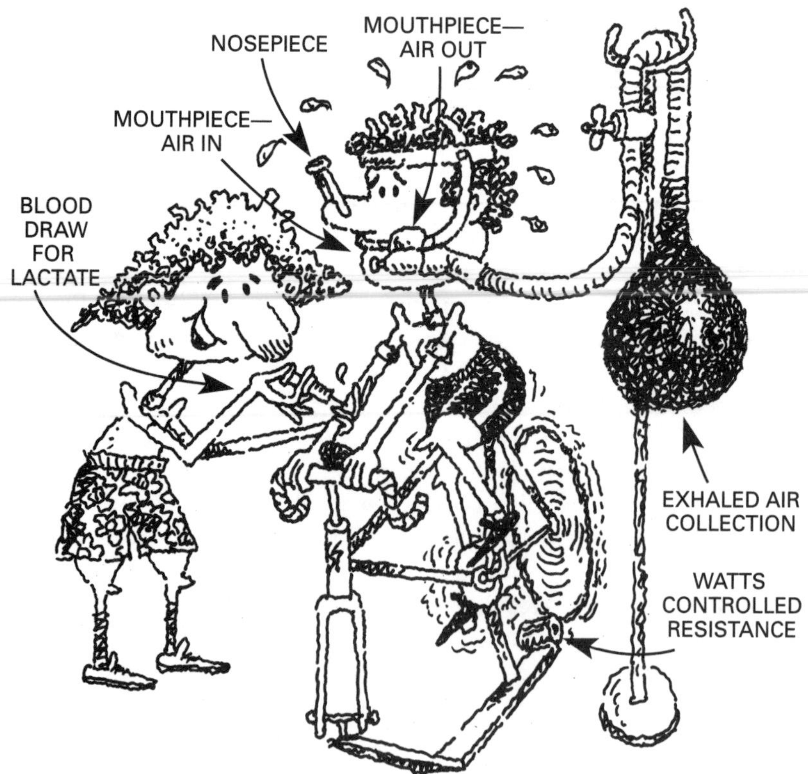

VO_2 max test

It is interesting, but not necessary, to measure the work that the subject is performing during the test. Workload can be determined on a treadmill if the speed and angle of the treadmill are known. Work can be determined on a bicycle ergometer—a specific type of stationary bicycle that measures power output. Power output is usually measured in watts.

It is interesting, but not necessary, to measure lactate levels in the blood at the same time. From this analysis, it is possible to gain insight into the anaerobic threshold, the maximum percentage of the maximum heart rate that can be maintained, and the economy or efficiency of the subject.

Limitations

This test is a measure of aerobic capacity. It doesn't give an indication of anaerobic power, muscle strength, tactical knowledge, or motivation. The test is a better predictor of athletic performance in some circumstances than in others. Some athletic situations have very good correlations with VO_2 max, e.g., running and bicycling uphill; some don't.

Flat time trials have more to do with power output and aerodynamics. Two riders with identical total oxygen use per minute, but different weights, will have different VO_2 max, but their air resistance may be similar. The rider with the higher VO_2 max will not be as much faster as might be expected on the basis of VO_2 max numbers alone. Weight is not as critical a factor in flat time trials.

VO_2 max does not measure economy of activity. Two cyclists may have identical VO_2 max values, but they may travel the same speed at different percentages of their VO_2 max. Two cyclists may have the same ability to use oxygen, but one may be able to use a higher fractional percentage over a prolonged time.

Here's a simple example: Suppose two athletes of the same shape and weight have identical VO_2 max. Suppose one athlete can ride a 40-K time trial at 93% of his maximum heart rate, but the other can maintain only 80%. The athlete who can ride at a higher percentage will be faster.

During the racing season, elite athletes may see their VO_2 max drop slightly—their muscle mass remains the same or drops slightly, while their economy improves—so cardiovascular demand is reduced. They will be able to perform the same or greater amounts of work, yet the amount of oxygen they must consume in order to perform this work is less.

Table 2-7 **VO_2 Max Values***

Group	VO_2 Max (mL/kg/m)
European pro tour winners, men	80+
U.S. Olympic Team, men	80
U.S. Cat 1, men	75
U.S. Cat 2, men	70
U.S. Cat 3, men	65
U.S. Cat 1, women	65
U.S. Cat 2–3, women	60
Elite masters women, age >40	50
College men, non-athletes	45
College women, non-athletes	40

* These are typical values as reported in the literature and from our own studies. Athletes may have numbers twice as high as those of sedentary persons.

Progressive Power Output

Determine Your Maximum Progressive Power Output

Perform this test with a device that measures power output, usually in watts. It can be performed in a lab, on a standard ergometer. It can also be performed at home. Several manufacturers make home stationary trainer devices that set power output, on which you mount your own bicycle. Although such home devices were once inaccurate, their validity is improving.

The power output you are looking for is the result of a progressive (ramped) aerobic effort lasting 10 to 16 minutes. It is not the peak power, which is supportable for only a few seconds and occurs after relative rest rather than after progressive aerobic effort.

I select one of a few different protocols, depending upon the expected fitness of the rider. For example, a masters, new-male, or seasoned-female racer might start out at 60 watts and progress 20 watts each minute until exhaustion. A professional athlete might start out at 60 watts, progress 40 watts each minute until 300 watts, and then progress 20 watts each minute until exhaustion.

Riders are given full credit for the 20-watt increment only if they can complete the entire minute stage. If they can complete 30 seconds, they are given

10 watts of credit. For example, a rider who completes a full minute of work at 220 watts, and 30 seconds at 240 watts, is considered to have performed 230 watts of work.

Rate Your Performance

As in the VO_2 max test described above, it's standard to divide output in watts by weight in kilograms. Divide weight in pounds by 2.2 to obtain weight in kilograms. For example, a rider who performs 230 watts of work and weighs 60 kg (132 pounds) has accomplished 3.8 watts per kilogram.

Table 2-8 **Watts per Kilogram Values***

Group	Watts/Kg
European pro tour winners, men	7.0+
U.S. Cat 1, men	6.0
U.S. Cat 2, men	5.5
U.S. Cat 3, men	5.2
U.S. Cat 1, women	5.2
U.S. Cat 2 – 3, women	4.7
Elite masters women, age >40	4.0
College men, non-athletes	3.5
College women, non-athletes	3.0

*These are typical values as reported in the literature and from our own studies. Athletes may have numbers twice as high as those of sedentary persons.

Predicting VO_2 Max from Bicycle Ergometry

It's much easier to be power tested on an ergometer than to have a true VO_2 max test with expired gas analysis performed in a physiology lab. It's also less expensive. An estimate of VO_2 max can be made simply from a knowledge of the power output and the weight of the subject.

I have devised the following formula:

$$VO_2 \text{ max (estimate)} = (\text{power in watts} \times 12 / \text{weight in kilograms} + 3.3$$
$$= (W \times 12 / kg) + 3.3$$

For example, consider a 154-pound (70 kg) rider who rides for 13 minutes, completing the 300-watt stage.

$$VO_2 \text{ max (estimate)} = (300 \times 12 / 70) + 3.3 = 54.7$$

Table 2-9 **Predicting VO_2 (mL/kg/min), from Progressive Bicycle Ergometry**

Exercise Power (watts)	Body Weight (pounds)				
	100	125	150	175	200
50	20	16	—	—	—
75	26	21	18	—	—
100	33	26	22	19	—
125	40	32	26	23	20
150	46	37	31	26	23
175	53	42	35	30	26
200	59	48	40	34	30
225	66	53	44	38	33
250	73	58	48	41	36
275	79	63	53	45	40
300	86	69	57	49	43
325	92	74	62	53	46
350	—	79	66	57	50
375	—	84	70	60	53
400	—	90	75	64	56
425	—	—	79	68	59
450	—	—	83	72	63
475	—	—	88	75	66

Power Output Is More Important Than VO_2 Max

The above formula implies a direct relationship between power output and VO_2 max. It is assumed that muscular energy and oxygen use go toward leg power. Occasionally, lab testing shows that riders may increase their power output but VO_2 max is unchanged or is even a little bit lower, or power stays the same and VO_2 max is reduced. The discrepancy between power output and VO_2 max relates to economy. For example, some cyclists are uneconomical, wasting energy in arm tension. As riding style improves, they become more economical. They are able to put out the same power with less oxygen use. It's not unusual for elite athletes to have increased leg power output but decreased VO_2 during the racing season because of improved economy.

Although maximum oxygen consumption (VO_2 max) is considered by many to be the most important physiological measure of an athlete's aerobic endurance potential, I prefer a progressive power test. It's power, not oxygen use, that gets an athlete down the road.

Submax Power and Submax Heart Rate

Here are a couple of other measures of fitness that are tested at the same time as maximum progressive power output. These measures of fitness are especially helpful in the repeated testing of the same individual to evaluate changes in fitness. I find these measures of fitness to be even better predictors of performance than VO_2 max and maximum progressive power output. In my experience, they are the most important testing markers available for road racers, time trialists, and mountain bikers.

SUBMAX POWER

Submax power can be defined in several ways. In physiology labs, submax power is determined as "power at threshold." An attempt is made to determine the lactate or other threshold. Power is measured at this intensity level. Although this is a common and accepted protocol, I believe this method is unnecessary, costly, and prone to added measurement errors. For more information about thresholds, see page 85.

I look at the power generated at 85% of an athlete's maximum heart rate. Since maximum heart rate may change in repeated testing, I look at the power output generated at the same heart rate as in the first test to evaluate changes in fitness.

SUBMAX HEART RATE

I look at heart rate response when the athlete finishes the stage that is closest to 75% of the maximum progressive power output. For example, I look at the heart rate at the end of the 240-watt stage of an athlete who completes 300 watts in a maximal progressive power output test. Since maximum progressive power output may change in repeated testing, I look at the heart rate at the same power output as determined in the first test to evaluate changes in fitness.

How Muscles Work

A basic understanding about how muscles work is important in understanding how the body responds to physical training.

Muscle Connections

A muscle is a contractile tissue. The two ends of a muscle form *ligaments,* which attach to bones. When a muscle contracts, it causes movement.

The Parts of a Muscle

Muscle is composed of smaller and smaller component parts. The component parts are covered and held together with connective tissue.

Figure 2-3

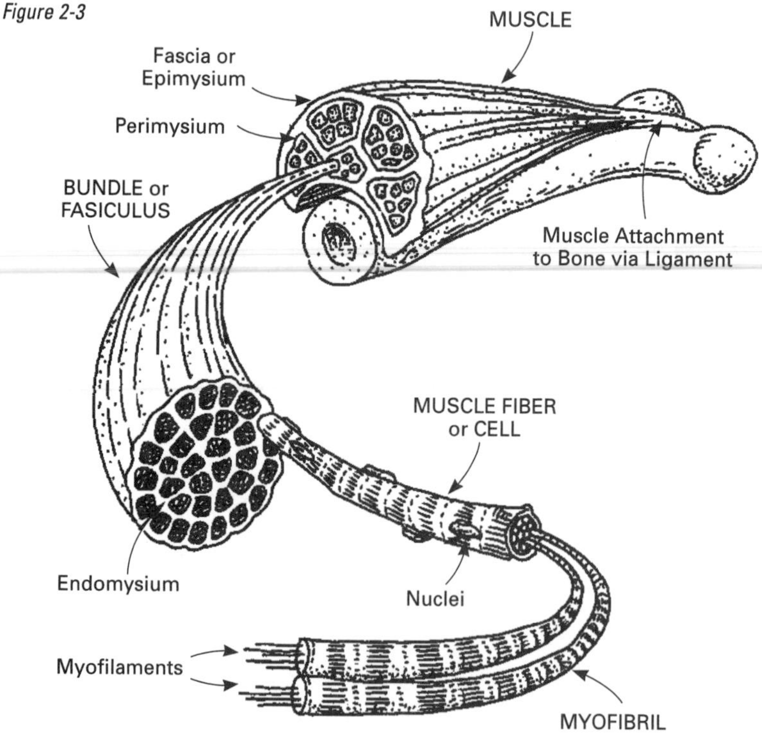

The parts of a muscle
(From D. R. Lamb, *The Physiology of Exercise: Responses and Adaptions,* 2d ed. Copyright © 1984 by Allyn & Bacon. Reprinted by permission.)

The overall connective tissue covering of a muscle is called the *fascia* or *epimysium.* Muscles are composed of bundles of *fibers.* A bundle of fibers is called a *fasciculus.* Each bundle is bound to neighboring fasiculi by connective tissue called *perimysium.* Each muscle fiber within each fasciculus is bound to others by connective tissue called *endomysium.* Each muscle fiber contains hundreds of contractile *myofibrils,* as well as the usual cellular apparatus such as nuclei and mitochondria.

Muscle Fiber Filaments

Each myofibril in turn contains many protein threads, called myofilaments. There are two types of filaments, thin filaments and thick filaments, as shown in Figure 2-4. Because the filaments are arranged in an organized and regular appearance, they appear as bands when observed under a microscope.

Figure 2-4

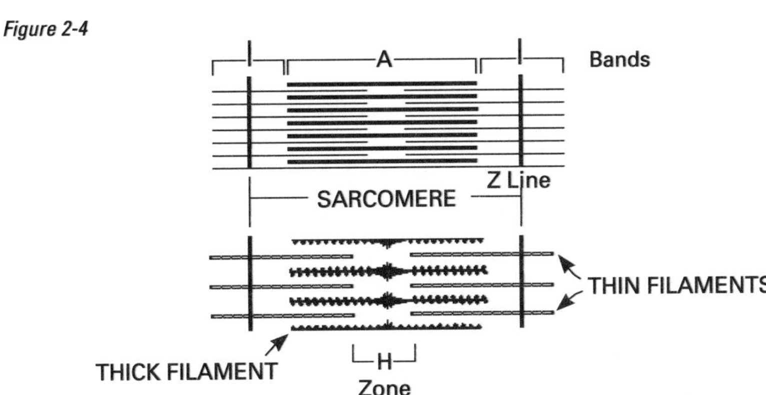

Muscle fiber filaments (schematic representations)

The dark bands, called *A bands,* are where the thin and thick filaments overlap. The light bands, called *I bands,* are only thin filaments. Each light band is bisected by a *Z line,* or disc, which appears to anchor the thin filaments. The distance between two Z lines is a *sarcomere.*

Cross-Bridges

The thin filaments contain the protein *actin.* The thick filaments contain the protein *myosin.* In the presence of these proteins, energy, and other substances, actin and myosin interact, forming connections, or *cross-bridges.* The interaction slides the filaments along each other, contracting the muscle. When the filaments are optimally overlapped, the number of cross-bridges is maximal, and the greatest contractile force can result. When the myofilaments are too far apart, or overlapped too much, less effective contraction results.

According to the cross-bridges theory, the optimal length of an isolated muscle to produce the maximum force of that muscle usually occurs when the muscle is slightly longer than its resting state.

Biomechanics

When dissected from the body and examined in the lab, muscles contract the most strongly when tested at lengths slightly longer than their resting states. In vivo, muscles attach to bones across joints. Their contraction results in movement of those joints. The force with which movement takes place relates not only to the intrinsic strength of the muscle but also to the leverage exerted by muscle across joints.

To understand this concept, consider arm wrestling on a table as a test of muscle strength. If two equally strong contestants compete, with their elbows placed equidistant from a perpendicular dropped to the table, it's a fair match. If contestants start with arms already halfway to the table, one will be at a disadvantage, the other advantaged.

Understanding the biomechanics of muscle function helps us understand why riders have more or less power in certain bicycle positions. Riders climb sitting upright, with their hands on the tops of the handlebars, because they have more power that way. They time trial bent over because improved aerodynamics more than compensate for the loss of power.

Muscle Types

Muscle fibers are adapted by heredity and activity for the work they perform. Muscle fibers are classified by the speed with which they contract to an electrical stimulus. *Slow-twitch,* or *Type I,* fibers respond relatively slowly, taking about 100 milliseconds to respond to a stimulus. *Fast-twitch,* or *Type II,* fibers respond more than twice as quickly, taking about 50 milliseconds to respond.

Different muscle groups have different percentages of fast-twitch fibers. The calf muscle, for example, is almost all slow-twitch. The eye muscles are almost all fast-twitch. Different people have different percentages of slow- and fast-twitch fibers in the same muscle groups. Some cyclists have 75% fast-twitch in their quads; some have 75% slow-twitch.

Slow-twitch fibers are more adapted to aerobic activity. They have more mitochondria, or energy factories, and a greater blood supply. Fast-twitch fibers are more adapted to anaerobic activity. They have more glycogen.

Table 2-10 **Characteristics of Fiber Types**

	Slow-Twitch	Fast-Twitch
Type	Type I	Type II
Response time	110 milliseconds	50 milliseconds
Size	Smaller	Larger
Force	Less overall force	More force
Efficiency	More energy efficient	Less energy efficient
Fatigability	Less fatigable	More fatigable
Mitochondria	More mitochondria	Fewer mitochondria
Blood supply	More capillaries	Fewer capillaries
Glycogen	Little glycogen	Lots of glycogen
Color stain	Red	White

Two Types of Fast-Twitch Fibers

Fast-twitch fibers are subdivided into two groups on the basis of their ability to produce energy. Type IIA can produce energy by aerobic and anaerobic metabolism; they are also known as fast oxidative glycolytic fibers (FOG). Type IIB fibers have few mitochondria and produce energy almost exclusively by anaerobic metabolism; they are also known as fast glycolytic fibers (FG). Both Type IIA and Type IIB fibers have large stores of glycogen for quick energy.

Fiber Types, Heredity, and Training

Although more research needs to be done in this area, it is believed that specific training tends to hypertrophy, or make larger, the fibers corresponding to the type of activity. It is not believed that the percentage of slow-twitch versus fast-twitch fibers changes.

Within Type II fibers, however, it is believed that the type may change from A to B in response to training. For example, muscle may adapt to anaerobic work by increasing the size of Type II fibers but not their total number. Response to anaerobic training may also shift Type IIB fibers to Type IIA.

Value of Fiber Typing

The major value of fiber typing is as a research tool. The realized development of most athletes in both aerobic and anaerobic activity usually relates more to training and motivation than to specific fiber percentages. Although some athletes are known for their excellence in sprinting or endurance, many others are excellent at both activities. Fiber typing can be a motivating factor, but it is just as likely to be used as an excuse for poor performance in a given event. As I said earlier when discussing genetic ability, I do not recommend fiber typing to athletes.

Muscle Fatigue

We all know the feeling of muscular fatigue. What causes fatigue and how can it be minimized?

What We're Talking About

Muscular fatigue is the inability to maintain or repeat the production of muscular force. It is different from muscle soreness, which is described on page 108.

Possible Causes

A muscle contracts because the brain—the highest center of the central nervous system—sends a signal down through the spinal cord to a peripheral nerve. This electrical signal is transmitted at a "junction box"—the neuromuscular junction—to the muscle. The electrical signal then stimulates the muscle to contract.

Table 2-11 **Possible Causes of Muscular Fatigue**

Location	Contribution to Fatigue
Central nervous system	Some
Peripheral nerve	None
Neuromuscular junction	Minimal
Muscle	Great

Theoretically, fatigue may occur from causes at any location from the brain down to the muscle. In fact, there is evidence that all of the above locations, with the exception of the peripheral nerve, can contribute to fatigue. In some cases, fatigue is due to a combination of factors.

THE CENTRAL NERVOUS SYSTEM

There are several reasons to think that the central nervous system contributes to fatigue:

- Muscles fatigued by voluntary muscle contractions can continue to respond to electrical stimulation.
- Mental activity—for example, cheering or performing arithmetic—affects endurance.
- Electrical activity, which originates from the central nervous system, changes with fatigue.
- Pain and motivation, although measured subjectively, are known to contribute to fatigue.

THE NEUROMUSCULAR JUNCTION

Limited electrical studies have shown that this nerve–muscle "junction box" may be related to muscular fatigue.

THE MUSCLE

This is believed to be the most likely cause of fatigue. The major causes are these:

- Depletion of the energy stores of adenosine triphosphate (ATP), creatine phosphate (CP), and glycogen
- Accumulation of lactic acid and other acidic products

Other factors that are associated with fatigue include:

- Percentage of fast-twitch fibers: The greater the percentage, the earlier the fatigue.
- Impaired release and accumulation of calcium in the transfer tubules of muscle cells; this problem is associated with reduced calcium availability and affects actin-myosin cross-bridging.

Muscle Causes of Fatigue Related to Duration of Activity

Activity up to 10 seconds. The rate of depletion of ATP and CP is believed to be important. It is thought that the making and breaking of actin-myosin cross-bridges occurs faster than energy can be supplied to keep them forming.

Activity from 10 seconds to 3 minutes. The depletion of ATP and CP is important, and the formation of lactic acid limits activity. Lactic acid lowers the blood pH, reducing the ability to form energy from glucose and preventing actin-myosin cross-bridging from occurring.

Activity from 3 to 15 minutes. Lactic acid becomes more important as a fatigue-limiting factor.

Activities from 15 minutes to 1 hour. A combination of lactic acid, glycogen depletion, and increase in body temperature may cause fatigue.

Activities from 1 to 4 hours. Glycogen depletion is the major factor. Dehydration may contribute to heat exhaustion.

How to Reduce Muscle Fatigue

The general training principles outlined in this book improve the body's adaptations to exertion.

Train specifically for the type of activity you wish to perform. For example, minimizing fatigue in sprint activities means improving the speed at which replenishment of ATP and CP occurs. This is accomplished by short intense efforts.

Exercise at an intensity level that produces lactic acid levels similar to those produced by the activities that require lactic acid tolerance.

Improve glycogen capacity for events of up to several hours' duration by not depleting glycogen in the two days preceding the event. Ingest sufficient carbohydrates to efficiently "fill up" the glycogen tank.

Strength Versus Power

Muscular Strength

Muscular strength is the greatest amount of force that a muscle can produce in a single maximal effort. It is usually assessed by noting the maximum force that a muscle can generate on a piece of weight-lifting equipment specially designed to accurately measure such force.

Strength is related to:

- Hypertrophy of muscle fibers
- Percentage of fibers within the muscle that are activated

Strength is proportional to the cross-sectional area of the muscle.

The number of muscle fibers is not believed to increase with training. Strength is related to the hypertrophy, or increase in size, of muscle fibers. In weight training, the strength phase of training is sometimes called the hypertrophy phase. That's a good name, because hypertrophy of muscle fibers is the single best predictor of strength performance. But it doesn't tell the whole story. At any given time, not all muscle fibers are activated. Studies have shown that the *percentage* of fibers that can be recruited increases with training.

Muscular Power

Muscular power is the product of force and speed. Since speed is distance per unit of time, muscular power may also be defined as the product of force and distance divided by time.

Power is related to

- Strength, i.e., hypertrophy of muscle fibers and the percentage of fibers within the muscle that are activated.
- Muscle cell energy production, including increased stores from creatine phosphate, ATP, and glycogen.
- Blood supply
- Lactic acid clearance and tolerance.
- Skill: Training improves economy as the increasing skill of the athlete results in fewer extraneous muscle contractions.

TYPES OF MUSCULAR POWER

Since power is defined as the product of force and distance divided by time, it is dependent upon the distance or time involved. Power may be any of several kinds:

- *Peak power:* The highest level of power achievable over a very short period of time, perhaps only a second or two. It is easy to measure. A bicycle ergometer is set up to read power output, usually in watts. The subject works as hard as possible to achieve the highest "instantaneous" number.
- *VO_2 Max power:* A bicycle ergometer is used. The subject follows an appropriate protocol with a graded increase in power output every minute. At some point the athlete can no longer maintain or increase power output. This value may range from one-eighth to one-half of peak power.
- *Threshold power:* An ergometer or power meter is used to monitor the athlete's power output during a time trial. What power level, for example, can an athlete maintain for a one-hour time trial? Whereas peak power is heavily dependent on fast-twitch fibers, threshold power is related to slow-twitch fibers.

Muscle Soreness

Three explanations for muscle soreness caused by exercise are often advanced. One appears to be correct. Strategies for minimizing muscle soreness are outlined.

What We're Talking About

Muscle soreness caused by exercise. It's different from muscle fatigue, which is discussed on page 104. Although exertion sometimes causes discomfort during exercise, we're talking about delayed onset muscle soreness (DOMS), which occurs from hours up to three days after activity.

Delayed muscle soreness is much more frequent in eccentric contractions than in concentric ones. Eccentric contractions are those that occur while the muscle is lengthening. This is especially interesting because eccentric contractions are easier to perform than concentric ones. It is easier to let oneself down slowly from a chin-up than it is to pull up—yet those who perform let-downs are more likely to be sore than those who perform chin-ups.

Three Possible Causes of Muscle Soreness

- Lactic acid
- Muscle spasm
- Tissue damage

Lactic Acid

Many articles written for athletes and some written for the general consumer still refer to this as a cause of delayed muscle soreness. But this is unlikely to be an explanation, because lactic acid is cleared from muscles within 30 minutes. Some activities associated with soreness produce no lactic acid. Some people who have diseases that prevent lactic acid from being formed still get sore. And soreness is more likely with eccentric contractions, which produce less lactic acid than concentric ones.

Muscle Spasm

According to this theory, lack of blood supply to the muscle causes the release of pain substances that trigger muscle spasms. Some support for this theory comes from electrical studies showing that sore muscles do have more electrical activity or spasm than those that are not sore. Also, stretching sometimes helps to relieve soreness and reduce electrical activity at the same time.

Since just stretching improperly can cause delayed muscle soreness, and is not associated with lack of blood supply or electrical activity, the muscle spasm theory is not likely to be a complete explanation.

Tissue Damage

This theory states that pain fibers are stimulated by swollen muscle tissue. Swelling in muscle tissue results from the release of chemicals from damaged or torn muscle fibers. This is the most likely and popular explanation for muscle soreness for these reasons:

- Microscopic fiber damage has been observed after activities associated with muscle soreness.
- Muscle-specific proteins have been found in the blood and urine of people who participate in strenuous activity.
- Those experiencing less muscle soreness have fewer of these muscle-specific proteins in the blood.
- The release of muscle enzymes into the blood is greater after eccentric exercise than after concentric exercise.

How to Reduce Muscle Soreness

Since soreness is more likely to occur from jerky eccentric movements, and since soreness occurs more often in those who begin a program after a period of inactivity:

- Begin with light activity, in both intensity and duration.
- Progressively and slowly increase intensity and duration.
- Avoid jerky, eccentric movements until you are well accustomed to the activity.

Efficiency and Economy

Efficiency and economy are important physiological measures of performance. They do not mean the same thing. Most of us use these terms imprecisely, and this causes confusion.

Efficiency

An athlete eats food to obtain calories for energy. The body metabolizes that food and, through chemical reactions, fuels the muscles to produce energy for work. Not all that goes into the body is used for energy production. The body's engine is not 100% efficient—much energy is wasted, or lost, in heat. In order to produce a given amount of work, the athlete must consume about four times as many calories as are produced.

Athletic efficiency is the amount of energy produced by an athlete, in calories, divided by the amount of energy metabolized by the athlete, in calories, to produce that work.

This measure has its origins in mechanical and engineering design. An engine might produce 500 watts of power. If the engine needs 2,000 watts (or the equivalent in gasoline or electricity) to drive it, then its efficiency is 25%. The loss of power is related to heat loss. When the human body is the engine being evaluated, the caloric equivalent of power is the measure often used. For example, to perform 25 calories of work, an individual might need to consume 100 calories.

Efficiency is a ratio. It is not a measure of the absolute calories used by the athlete. Intuitively, most of us think of efficiency as a good quality. This is not necessarily so for the athlete. Since athletes are more inefficient when burning fats than when burning carbohydrates, and since sparing glycogen is good, elite athletes may be less efficient at burning fuels than untrained subjects.

Economy

Economy can also be related to mechanics. It is defined as the energy expenditure required for a given workload. It can apply to heart rate, oxygen consumption, or calories.

Here's an example of economy: An athlete has a maximum heart rate of 180 beats per minute. At a certain speed she has a heart rate of 160. After training, at the same speed, she has a heart rate of 155. Economy has improved.

Or, consider two athletes who have the same VO_2 max. One can cycle at 200 watts using 80% of VO_2 max. The other, cycling at the same power, requires 85% of VO_2 max. The first athlete's energy expenditure is more economical.

RELATING EFFICIENCY AND ECONOMY

To ride at a certain speed, athlete A's muscles perform 25 calories of work per unit time and metabolize 100 calories to do so (75 calories are inefficiently lost to heat). Athlete B's muscles perform 30 calories of work at the same speed and metabolize 105 calories to do so. Athlete A: 25 /100. Athlete B: 30 /105.

- The efficiency of athlete A is 25/100, or 25%. The efficiency of athlete B is 30/105, or 28.6%. Athlete B is more efficient.
- The economy of athlete A is better. Fewer calories are needed to travel at the same speed.

Training improves economy. It may worsen efficiency.

Optimal Cadence

Determining the optimal pedaling frequency is not easy. Several studies have examined this question, but they do not necessarily point the way for training recommendations.

What We're Talking About

We're discussing the best cadence, or pedaling frequency. There is no single best pedaling frequency. The best cadence depends upon the individual rider and the type of riding. Most racers prefer a cadence between 80 and 110 r.p.m. They ride at a lower cadence in time trials, and a higher cadence in criteriums or mass start track events.

Studies have found relationships between cadence and efficiency and economy. Whether these studies have any practical importance is controversial.

Optimal Cadence and Efficiency

Most cadence studies have examined the relationships among cadence, power output, and efficiency on bicycle ergometers. Efficiency, as discussed previously, is calculated by measuring calories used per unit of time to maintain a power output. These studies show that a cadence much below that normally preferred by racers is the most efficient.

As power output rises, optimal pedaling rate often increases. Although there is a change in optimal cadence depending upon the power level examined, almost all studies have shown that the most efficient cadence is still well below 80 r.p.m. Some studies have shown optimal values in the low 30s.

Optimal Cadence and Economy

Cadence can also be examined in relation to economy rather than efficiency. For example, at a specified work load, one can determine what cadence results in the lowest oxygen consumption or lowest heart rate. Such studies performed on a bicycle ergometer also show that optimal pedaling frequency is lower than most racers prefer.

Problems Relating Cadence to Efficiency or Economy

PROBLEM 1

Tests that look at caloric consumption, heart rate, or oxygen consumption ignore the importance of muscle fatigability and endurance. Sure, it's true that at any given speed, the bigger the gear, the lower the heart rate. The problem is that the lower the cadence, the more fast-twitch muscle fibers are recruited. (Most people guess incorrectly that "faster cadences" are associated with more "fast-twitch" muscle fiber recruitment, perhaps because the word "fast" appears in both phrases. For the same speed, however, there is more muscle tension at slower cadences, and more recruitment of fast-twitch fibers.) The more fast-twitch muscle fibers are recruited, the greater the production of lactic acid. Racers know that muscle fatigue often limits performance—riding in too big a gear is great for saving cardiovascular effort, but the legs bog down, lug, and quit.

PROBLEM 2

Bicycle ergometer tests are not applicable to real-world riding. A flat, windless time trial is pretty close to the steady-state power work one examines on an ergometer. Even the best time trial courses have undulations or passing trucks. Big gears make responding to these relatively small fluctuations in speed extra fatiguing and taxing.

And that's for time trials. Criteriums are even more extreme, with frequent jumps through corners. It's common for a rider who time trials in a 53/13 gear to ride a criterium in a 53/16.. That's a difference in cadence of 20 to 25 r.p.m.

Cycling on the road or track, on a freely moving bicycle, involves changes in inertial forces and the center of gravity that are different than on stationary ergometers. When bicycles are ridden on treadmills, rather than on stationary ergometers, optimal cadence is determined to be closer to the higher cadences cyclists prefer.

The optimal cadence determined by any test on an ergometer is the optimal cadence for riding an ergometer, not for real-world riding.

PROBLEM 3

Bicycle ergometer testing of optimal cadence usually does not account for perceived exertion. (A problem is that perceived exertion is very difficult to quantify and measure.) Athletes may select gears related to perceived exertion rather than their caloric or oxygen consumption, heart rates, or other factors. Unless motivated by perceived training needs, riders are basically lazy—by which I mean that their bodies naturally try to accomplish work in the "easiest" manner. Since higher cadences are associated with reduced pedal forces, perceived exertion may be lower.

Perceived exertion also depends upon the athlete's state of recovery. For example, riders may climb the same hill at a certain cadence on a day when they are fresh and at a faster cadence when they are tired, even though they ride both days at the same speed.

PROBLEM 4

Once riders have already adapted to a "suboptimal" position, testing in various other configurations may not reveal the true advantage of the "optimal" position until they have had time to adapt.

MEDICAL PROBLEMS

At a higher power output, big-gear riding is harder on the musculoskeletal system, causing more muscle soreness and more joint pains. Empirically, big-gear riding results in a greater risk of injury.

Arnie's Optimal Cadence Determination

Here's one method I use for advising riders on their optimal cadence in time trialing. I use an electronic stationary trainer. This allows the athlete's own bicycle to be used on an ergometer, on which resistance can be set at any wattage value. No matter what cadence or gear the athlete selects, the same power level is required to turn the cranks.

I perform the test by increasing the resistance level by 20 watts each minute and recording cadence at each level. At some point, the athlete can no longer continue. Cadence and heart rate fall, and the athlete is exhausted.

The athlete has self-selected a cadence for any given power level. Since most athletes time trial at about 90% of maximum heart rate, we use the cadence level recorded when the athlete reached this level as a starting point in actual road time-trial testing. We then use the results of actual tests to further refine the optimal cadence.

Cadence Summary

Lab studies of physiology have looked at optimal cadence. These studies have confirmed that for a given speed, bigger gears and slower r.p.m. improve efficiency and lower oxygen consumption and heart rate. But physiological or mechanical efficiency is not what is important here. These studies ignore muscle fatigability, endurance, perceived effort, and the changing pace of real-world riding. Each rider's optimal cadence is specific to that rider. No matter what the studies say, you've got to find your own.

Optimal Crankarm Length

Determining the optimal crankarm length is not easy. Several studies have examined this question, but they do not help in training recommendations.

What We're Talking About

The optimal length of the crankarms. It depends upon the athlete's anatomy, the type of riding, training, and adaptation.

When I first took up track racing, I observed many different crankarm lengths on the bicycles at the velodrome. Crankarm lengths of 165 millimeters were common. Some riders rode 167.5-millimeter crankarm, some 170-millimeter. For kilometer and pursuit races I saw 172.5-millimeter and occasionally 175-millimeter crankarms. I asked riders why they rode a certain length crankarm. The most common answer was "That's the way the bike came." There must be more to it than that, I thought.

Force and Optimal Crankarm Length

Archimedes had a physics lesson for us when he said, "Give me a lever long enough and I will move the world."

Studies of physiology have examined the force required to maintain a given bicycle speed. Not surprisingly, less force is required to turn the cranks when crankarm length is increased. Since the given bicycle speed is constant, and the gearing hasn't changed, the cadence remains the same. Many coaches and authors have mistakenly concluded that the power requirements with longer cranks are also reduced.

Power is the time rate of doing work. In a straight direction, power is the force applied times the velocity of the body to which the force is applied. Some have reasoned that the power required drops, since longer cranks reduce the force required.

But cranks rotate; they do not move in a straight line. This requires torque, which is force times the perpendicular distance from axis to line of action of force. In other words, when the crankarm length is longer, the torque required is greater for any constant force. The required force may be less, but the legs have to travel farther around a larger circle, requiring more torque, so we're back where we began. The bottom line is that the same studies that show a reduction in force with longer cranks also show that *the power requirement does not change.*

Examining power does not help us decide optimal crankarm length. In order to better study optimal crankarm length, we must study not only the forces involved but also muscle fatigability, heart rate, and oxygen consumption. I am not aware of any published studies that examine these variables.

Biomechanics and Optimal Crankarm Length

As discussed in the chapter "How Muscles Work" on page 100, muscles have an optimal angle of function. Although longer crankarms have been traditionally favored by time-trialists, it's easy to show that in the aero position longer cranks mean that knees rise higher, and hence closer to the chest—a worse angle of function. This results in reduced muscle power at the top of the stroke.

Acceleration and Optimal Crankarm Length

Conventional wisdom has it that shorter crankarms accelerate more quickly. This opinion is not universal. BMX riders traditionally use long crankarms. Many riders report that longer crankarms accelerate more quickly but that high r.p.m. cannot be maintained.

DETERMINE YOUR CRANKARM LENGTH

Although the science above may help, what we're still left with is empiricism, conventional wisdom, and trial and error.

Here are some guidelines:

- Crankarm length should be longer for taller riders. Height is related to inseam or leg length. Inseam or leg length is closer to what's important than height. The length of the femur, or thigh, is even closer. As most riders know or can measure their inseams easily, recommendations will be based on inseam.
- Shorter crankarms are preferred for quick acceleration events—mass start track races and criteriums. Track riders often must limit the length of their crankarms to avoid hitting the upper banked surface of the velodrome when they turn or lean their bicycles. Small frames often require short crankarms to avoid hitting the front wheel when turning.
- Longer cranks may be more suitable for steady riding such as time trials or climbing, including mountain biking.

Start with this: For riders with an inseam less than 31 inches, start with 170-millimeter cranks. Riders with an inseam of 31 or 32 inches use 172.5-millimeter cranks. Riders with an inseam over 33 inches use 175-millimeter cranks.

Modify with this: Track riders go down 2.5 or 5 millimeters in size. Time trialists go up 2.5 millimeters; mountain bikers go up 5 millimeters.

Caution: Once you have used one crankarm length for a while, modifying the length more than 2.5 millimeters at a time is not recommended. Although another length may be advantageous in the long run, your body, having adapted to the current length, will take time to readapt and become economical at a new length. Changes in crankarm length more than 2.5 millimeters at a time may also make you more prone to injury.

Crankarm Summary

Lab studies of physiology have looked at optimal crankarm length. These studies have confirmed that for a given speed, longer cranks require less force. But your legs need to go faster, and power requirements stay the same. Most studies have been too short, considering the relatively long time riders have adapted to their chosen crankarm length. The issues are complex. Other factors, such as frame construction and performance characteristics, may also be relevant. Studies don't help us enough in making real-world decisions. Conventional coaching wisdom and recommendations have been outlined here, but they are not based on a solid footing.

Putting It All Together: Efficiency, Cadence, and Crank Length

Despite the lack of good laboratory data, real-world bicycling recommendations can be made on the basis of known physical principles.

What We're Talking About

Putting together information regarding the efficiency and economy of cycling with recommendations or observations about cadence and crankarm length.

Lessons from Cars and Weight Lifting

Two real-world lessons make our thinking clearer.

LESSON 1

Imagine traveling a country road in a car at about 45 miles per hour. You're traveling in fifth gear, which is your most efficient in terms of gas consumption. The road is a little twisty, and you come upon another vehicle. You want to pass quickly to avoid an oncoming car. Down-shift to fourth. Your acceleration around the car ahead of you will be quicker.

LESSON 2

Consider weight lifting, say bench pressing. You could lift a very light weight, say half a pound, very quickly, or you could lift a heavy weight slowly. The heavy weight requires more strength, or force. The heaviest weight you can lift, just once, demonstrates your maximum strength. But it does not demonstrate your power. Power is force per unit of time.

Suppose the question is this: how much weight can you lift in one hour? Choose a weight and multiply it by the number of repetitions you can accomplish in one hour. Very heavy weights won't work, because you won't be able to lift them quickly, and your muscles will fatigue quickly. Very light weights won't work, because you'll not be able to lift them fast enough to compensate for their lightness. Clearly, the correct answer lies somewhere in between.

Some Conclusions

Optimal cadence depends on activity. Time trialists and mountain bikers will use a lower cadence than criterium riders,who, like the passing auto in Lesson 1 above, need snappier accelerations and higher r.p.m.

From Lesson 2, one can more clearly understand that optimal cadence is a balance between aerobic fitness and muscular fatigue. When one lacks aerobic fitness, one compensates by pushing a bigger gear. When one lacks strength, one compensates by using smaller gears.

An athlete might time trial at high altitude in a bigger gear with a slower cadence than at sea level because the reduced pressure of oxygen in the air reduces aerobic capacity.

Shorter cranks, which travel in smaller circles, can be turned faster. They are more suitable for acceleration and high r.p.m. events like track sprints and criteriums. Longer cranks may require less perceived force for the same power output and are more suitable for time trials.

Optimal crank length and cadence are dependent upon a person's anatomy and training adaptations.

Optimal Pedal Stroke

What We're Talking About

What is the most effective way to pedal a bicycle? Should one concentrate on pushing down, or forward? Is it important to pull up with the leg? Is the technique of ankling—changing the foot position at the ankle while pedaling—effective?

What We Know

Elite and non-elite cyclists have been studied using force-measuring pedals and computer video analysis. Pulling-through and pulling-up forces were once thought to be significant. However, re-examination of the data and subtraction of the inertial forces of the legs has shown that these forces are not as strong as was formerly believed. Elite cyclists are more effective because of greater downward forces, rather than because they unweigh their pedals or pull up more than recreational cyclists. Although some coaches strongly believe that specific pedal-style training improves performance, this has not been scientifically shown.

Optimal Seat Height

Seat height is a compromise between aerobic economy, aerodynamics, bicycle handling, injury prevention, muscle fatigue, stroke fluidity, and power.

Traditional Methods

You must not be so far extended that your hips rock or that your spin is restricted when you pedal. Some riders determine position by raising the seat until their heels can just clear the pedals. Traditional formulas based upon inseam measurements or other body dimensions can give only approximate results. They provide rough starting points. Cleat thickness, pedal type, seat type, and seat-tube angle all influence this form of measurement and must additionally be factored into any equation.

Optimal Method—Knee Angles

A better starting point is to base the seat height on the angle from the horizontal formed by the knee at the bottom of the pedal stroke. This angle is measured in degrees of flexion. With the lower leg extended straight out, this angle is zero degrees by convention. As a starting point, many racers are best positioned so that the angle of the knee is 25 degrees. This is a good compromise between aerobic economy, muscle fatigue, stroke fluidity, and power.

I feel that athletes can often self-select their optimal leg extension. A favorite method of mine is to watch riders as they climb out of the saddle and to note the knee angle. I fix seat height so that the same knee angle is produced when they are seated.

Adjustments to Seat Height

Aerobic economy and power can be improved with a higher position: a knee angle of 15 to 20 degrees. This is important, for example, in climbing and time trialing. I believe that most athletes self-select their optimal knee extension for performance when climbing out of the saddle. I believe that performance is optimized when the seat height is adjusted to provide this same knee extension while the rider is seated.

More control can be obtained with a lower position: a knee angle of 30 degrees. This is important, for example, when riding a bicycle on a steep velodrome.

Riders with pain in the anterior (front) knee—due, for example, to arthritis or patellar tendonitis—do better with a higher seat position and a knee angle of 15 to 20 degrees. Riders with pain in the posterior (back) knee, in the Achilles tendon, or in the back of the calf or thigh do better with a lower seat position and a knee angle of 25 to 35 degrees.

Different individuals with the same leg lengths may differ in the flexibility and length of their muscles. Riders who stretch or have massage, especially "myofascial release" bodywork, may be able to ride with higher seat heights and more power.

Corrections and adjustments for individuals with different leg lengths are discussed in "Leg-Length Discrepancy" on page 209.

Measuring Body Fat

Body fat percentage is an important determinant of success as an athlete. There are advantages and disadvantages among the methods available for measuring it.

Why Measure Body Fat?

Stepping on the scale is a crude way to figure out how fat or thin you are. Consider two people who both weigh 150 pounds. One may have denser, or heavier, bones and more muscle than the other. The two will not have the same percentage of body fat. Other things being equal, the one with less fat will perform better. Leanness improves athletic performance on a bicycle, but excessive leanness is not necessarily healthy.

Table 2-12 **Body Fat Guidelines (%)**

	Men	Women
Elite athletes	5–10	10–15
Good, healthy	10–15	15–20
Fat restricts performance	15–20	20–25
Unhealthy	>20	>30
U.S. averages		
Under age 30	20	25
Over age 30	25	31

Many Methods for Measuring Body Fat

There are many ways to measure body fat. They include:

- Skin calipers
- Underwater (hydrostatic) weighing
- Electrical impedance
- Ultrasound
- Infrared light
- Computerized imaging

Factors to Consider

There are four factors to consider when measuring body fat:

- Validity or accuracy. Does the test measure what it is supposed to?
- Reliability or repeatability. How close are repeated measurements?
- Cost.
- Convenience.

Skin Calipers

This is the least expensive and most convenient method. Calipers are generally accurate to plus or minus 4% of true body fat percentage. The thickness of the skin and the subcutaneous (under-the-skin) fat is measured, usually at several locations. Based on these measurements, an estimate is made of body fat percentage.

Figure 2-5

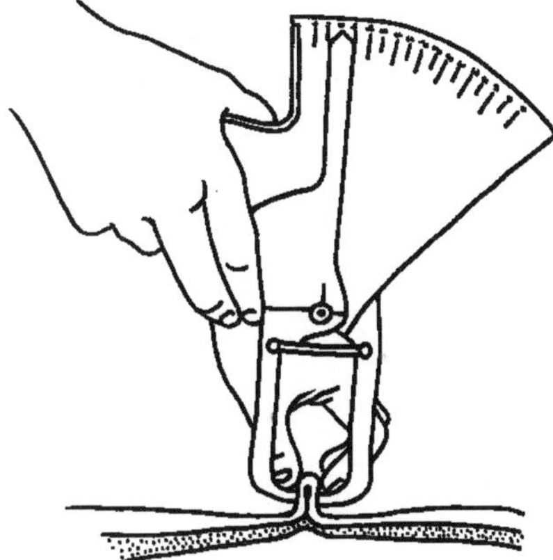

Using skin calipers to measure body fat

From one to twelve locations are measured. It is important to measure the correct anatomic site and to make sure the edges of the caliper have uniform and appropriate pressure when the skin and fat are being compressed. In general, the more locations measured, the more accurate the test. Reliability is dependent upon using the same tester.

Various assumptions are made about the distribution of fat in men and women. For this and other reasons, the sites measured differ in men and women.

One of the simplest ways to use skin calipers is to measure the skin thickness in three locations, add up the measurements, and consult a table that gives figures based upon age. Alternatively, a formula may be used to attach more or less value to the measurements at different sites.

Calipers can be purchased for as little as $10. More expensive calipers, costing hundreds of dollars, are sturdier and have better springs to exert uniform pressure during measurement. Expensive calipers may also have small, built-in computers with preprogrammed formulas for measuring different anatomic sites, attach relative values to those sites, and automatically read out body fat percentage for men and women of different ages.

Underwater Weighing

This is the "gold standard," perhaps the most accurate method.

Archimedes had it right years ago when he discovered that by weighing objects in water he could determine their density. As we all know, fatter people float more easily. By using Archimedes' principle and some other assumptions, one can use a scale and a large tank of water to determine body fat percentage. This method is less dependent upon the skill of the operator than skin calipers. Underwater weighing requires the athlete to exhale and hold the breath under water. The tank must be large enough to hold the athlete. Such tanks require significant physical space and are expensive. Although many university physiology labs have them, getting weighed underwater requires considerably more logistics than the use of calipers.

Determining the density of the athlete requires that the volume of air within the subject be excluded in the calculation of the volume of the athlete. For this reason, the athlete exhales before being weighed. But there is still residual air in the lungs, as well as a small amount of air in the bowels. The residual lung volume can be measured separately, and the amount of air in the bowels is given an assumed volume. If the amount of air remaining in the athlete's lungs is not measured separately but assumed on the basis of sex and age, the test is less accurate.

If the subject is able to empty the lungs of air well, and if the mathematical assumptions used by the operator are good ones, this is probably the most accurate method of determining body fat.

The first research into body fat percentage was performed with underwater weighing tests and correlated with autopsy studies of white men. The assumptions and formulas are most confidently extrapolated to white men. It is less certain that this test is as accurate for women and for non-white individuals.

Electrical Impedance

Fat and muscle conduct electricity differently. By measuring changes in electrical activity with safe, low currents, it is possible to estimate body fat percentage. This method does not require as much skill from the operator as skin calipers do. It is no more accurate than skin calipers, requires an expensive machine, and is not as commonly used as the above methods.

Ultrasound

Sound waves are reflected differently from fat than from muscle. By measuring the time it takes for sound waves to travel through fat to muscle and bounce back, it is possible to estimate body fat percentage. Like electrical impedance, this method does not require as much skill from the operator as skin calipers do, is no more accurate than skin calipers, and requires an expensive machine. It is not as commonly used as calipers and underwater weighing.

Infrared

Infrared light waves measure the distance across the fat layers under the skin. By use of these measurements and assumptions about the distribution of fats, the body fat percentage is calculated in a manner similar to the caliper method. Like electrical impedance and ultrasound, infrared does not require as much operator skill as skin calipers, is no more accurate than skin calipers, and requires an expensive machine. It is not as commonly used as calipers and underwater weighing.

Computerized Imaging

Modern radiological tools such as magnetic resonance imaging can be used, at great expense, to accurately measure body fat. This is an emerging technology.

Travel and Climate Problems

The body's acclimatization to a new geographic environment may represent a trivial adaptation. Occasionally, it can be extreme and life-threatening. Common travel and climate effects include:

- Time zone
- Cold
- Heat and humidity
- Altitude

General Advice

Increasing complex carbohydrates and reducing fat and protein consumption may be helpful. Avoid caffeine, alcohol, and simple carbohydrates. Heavy persons may have more problems with acclimatization than those who have low body fat percentages.

Time Zone Change

It is usually easier to travel west to east than east to west. Crossing one or two time zones usually presents no significant problem. Crossing three or four time zones presents challenges, and crossing five or more time zones requires at least several days for adaptation.

You can partially pre-adapt by rising an hour or two earlier or later, and retiring an hour or two earlier or later, depending upon whether you are traveling east or west.

Some riders keep their watches on home time. This is a mistake. It is important to set your watch to the new time zone when you arrive. It helps you physiologically adapt to the new time and helps prevent you from missing race start times.

Travel tends to make most people tired. Travel is hard work. Don't worry if you miss a day or two of training. If you cross many time zones, try to "stay up" and go to bed at the "right time" in the new time zone. A sleeping pill may help readjust your "internal clock" when used for a day or two. It often takes one day for each time zone crossed before you can feel and perform at your potential.

Cold

Muscles have an optimal operating temperature. Warmup helps them reach this level. Cold-weather riding makes it difficult for muscles to function well.

Tights and other protective gear can help performance significantly. Most riders perform better with tights when the temperature drops below 65°F on cloudy days or 60°F on sunny days. A thin layer protecting you against wind chill is often all you need. Wind-shell jackets, long-fingered gloves, and headbands are also useful as the temperature falls.

Since cold weather decreases muscle performance and work, it also results in a lower VO_2 max and lower heart rate.

Other things being equal, cold air is denser than warm air: Aerodynamics are worse, and the result is slower speeds. (However, when an advancing cold front is associated with a low-pressure system, speeds may be faster.)

A 20°F drop in air temperature results in about a one-minute increase in time-trial time per hour.

Heat and Cycling

What We're Talking About

How heat affects cycling performance and causes heat illness, and how heat's effects can be minimized. This is especially important to racers of long hilly road races that last a couple of hours or more.

Sweating

Sure, when it's hot we sweat. Blood flow to the skin helps shunt heat from the body's core. But it's not really sweating that cools so much as evaporation of the sweat. That's why tail-wind climbs are so hellacious in hot and humid conditions. A good head wind will slow you down but help keep you cool.

How Heat Affects Performance—Positives and Negatives

- Heat normally decreases the time necessary for warmup.
- Heat and humidity increase sweating, which increases dehydration and decreases performance.

- Heat increases the heart rate for a given workload, increases maximum heart rate, and decreases endurance cycling performance.
- Heat increases demands placed on the body—metabolism is speeded up and blood is shunted to the skin—so less energy is available for working muscles.
- Other things being equal, hot air is less dense, so time trial times may improve; when, however, heat is associated with a high-pressure weather system, time trial times may be worse because of increased air density.
- Drugs and alcohol may worsen the body's ability to tolerate heat, as do beta-blockers and diuretics (used for high blood pressure), antihistamines, and sedatives.

How Much Fluid Can One Lose?

In conditions of high heat and humidity, a maximum of up to a gallon an hour may be lost at high exertion levels. That represents a water bottle every seven or eight minutes! Most of the time, fluid loss is less than the maximum. Normally, a bottle every 15 to 20 minutes is sufficient. You can estimate fluid loss by weighing yourself before and after rides. A pint of water (16 ounces—a water bottle) weighs about a pound.

Fluid loss sets up a vicious circle. When you are hot you need to sweat more. But when you are dehydrated, you sweat less. When you sweat less, you can't get rid of body heat.

The sensation of thirst means you are already dehydrated. Drink before you are thirsty!

What About Electrolytes?

The major electrolyte lost in sweat is sodium. One teaspoon of salt may be lost with each quart of sweat. Potassium, magnesium, and chloride are also lost, but they are usually not a problem.

Most daily diets contain enough sodium to replace the losses in five quarts of sweat. On hot and humid days, ⅓ to ½ teaspoon of salt per water bottle helps replace the lost sodium and stimulates your thirst to keep you drinking. Although you can add the salt to your favorite drink or water, the palatability will probably be poor. Some commercial sports drinks, relatively high in sodium, will most likely work better. As always, experiment during training, not during a race.

Heat Illnesses

There are four major heat-related medical problems: heat cramps, heat exhaustion, exertional heat injury, and heat stroke. These are discussed in order of severity, starting with the least severe. Elements of more than one problem may be present at the same time. Exertional heat injury and heat stroke require emergency medical care.

HEAT CRAMPS

It's believed that an imbalance in the body's fluids and electrolytes contributes to this problem.

Treatment: Acclimatization, fluids, and salt may help.

HEAT EXHAUSTION

Weak rapid pulse, low blood pressure, headache, dizziness, weakness. Sweating may be reduced. Body temperature is not elevated to dangerous levels.

Treatment: Stop exercising. Move to a cooler environment. Sponge with water. Drink.

EXERTIONAL HEAT INJURY

Gooseflesh, sensation of chilling, throbbing headache, weakness, perhaps dry skin, nausea, vomiting, unsteady gait, incoherent speech, loss of consciousness.

Treatment: Stop exercising. Move to cooler environment. Sponge with cool water or ice. Cool showers or baths. Fans. Drink.

HEAT STROKE

Mental confusion, convulsions, loss of consciousness, increased body temperature. Sweating may stop; the skin may be dry and hot. Untreated, this condition may lead to death.

Treatment: Emergency treatment is required. Aggressive lowering of body temperature is required. Stop exercising. Move to air-conditioned environment. Take a cool shower or an ice bath. Fans. Chilled intravenous fluids.

Humidity and the Heat Stress Index

Humidity, which slows evaporation, makes temperatures seem hotter. Just as the wind-chill index accounts for the perceived lowering of temperature because of the interaction of wind and cold, the heat stress index takes into consideration the effect of humidity on perceived heat. This index can help us assess training risks when it's hot and humid.

Table 2-13 **Heat Stress Index**

Air Temperature in Degrees Fahrenheit	70	75	80	85	90	95	100	105	110	115	120
% Humidity											
0	64	69	73	78	83	87	91	95	99	103	107
10	65	70	75	80	85	90	95	100	105	111	116
20	66	72	77	82	87	93	99	105	112	120	130
30	67	73	78	84	90	96	104	113	123	135	148
40	68	74	79	86	93	101	110	123	137	151	
50	69	75	81	88	96	107	120	135	150		
60	70	76	83	90	100	114	132	149			
70	70	77	85	93	106	124	144				
80	71	78	86	97	113	136					
90	71	79	88	102	122						
100	72	80	91	108							

For example, if the temperature is 90 degrees and the humidity is 70%, the heat stress index is 106. Heat stress index readings of 90 to 105 are associated with heat cramps. Readings of 105 to 130 mean that heat cramps or heat exhaustion is likely. Exertional heat injury or heat stroke is possible. Above a heat stress index of 130, heatstroke is a definite risk.

Acclimatization

The body can adapt to hot and humid environments. Adaptation takes one to two weeks. Age and gender are not significant factors, but adaptation is harder for obese people.

The first workouts in the heat and humidity should be light. Even after several days of acclimatization, workouts should not be performed at maximum intensity. Even if you are not training at maximum, expect your body to demand more fluids than usual. Drink more.

If you are planning to compete or ride in a hot and humid environment, acclimatization before arrival may be helped by

- Wearing additional clothing
- Saunas, steam baths, and hot tubs

WHAT ACCLIMATIZATION DOES

- Improves blood flow to the skin
- Lowers threshold for the start of sweating
- Increases sweat output
- Lowers the salt concentration of sweat

Coping with Heat and Humidity

- Hydrate well before, during, and after riding.
- Increase your intake of fluids and salt.
- Wear light-colored clothing.
- Wear less clothing where clothing limits evaporation.
- Drink cool fluids with calories and salt.
- Sponge, spray, or pour water (preferably chilled) over your helmet, clothes, or body.
- Use sunscreen, but avoid waterproof nonbreathing types.
- Trim long hair; shave beard.
- Wear a well-ventilated helmet.
- Aspirin may help headache and possibly reduce body temperature.
- Specialty back packs loaded with ice may help.
- Consult your physician: Consider reducing use of some medicines, especially those for high blood pressure.

Performance with Heat and Humidity

Adaptations allow improved physical performance, but this improved performance is never as good in tropical conditions as it is in moderate climates.

Muscles have an optimal operating temperature. Exercise generates body heat. Hot bodies don't perform as well. The body cools itself through sweating. When the body is hot, more blood flows to the skin to aid in sweating, and less is available for your muscles. This decreases muscle performance and work. Dehydration is also more likely, and this in turn decreases performance.

Short efforts are not likely to be hindered by heat and humidity. Events longer than five minutes will be affected.

Altitude and Hypoxia

It's agreed that altitude acclimatization is helpful for athletes who wish to compete at altitude (above 7,000 feet). The use of altitude for the enhancement of sea-level performance is a hot topic among elite and professional coaches. Altitude training may or may not be that effective in improving human sea-level performance. Altitude "resting" may be a giant help.

Altitude—What We're Talking About

From the athletes' point of view, it means less oxygen—hypoxia. As one ascends to altitude, there's less barometric pressure; as a result, less oxygen is absorbed into the blood.

At sea level, the average barometric pressure is 760 millimeters of mercury. At 10,000 feet, the barometer reads 510. The percentage of oxygen in the air, about 21%, does not change—but the density of air, and hence oxygen, does. At 10,000 feet, only two-thirds of sea-level oxygen is present.

Side Effects—Altitude Sickness

Many who travel to altitude experience side effects. Most people adapt to altitude more quickly when they have traveled to altitudes frequently in the past. The side effects, however, are not predictable. Some individuals may have problems on some occasions and not on others. Problems do occur in proportion to the change in altitude. Those living at sea level have more problems when traveling to 8,000 feet than those living at 3,000 feet. Changes in altitude less than 4,000 feet do not present much difficulty.

Those who travel to 8,000 feet and above may experience headache, drowsiness, mental fatigue, dizziness, nausea, vomiting, insomnia, dimness of vision (especially color vision), and euphoria. Judgment and memory are ordinarily normal to 9,000 feet. At 11,000 feet, reaction times, handwriting, and psychological test scores may be 20% below normal. Pulmonary edema, convulsions, and coma can occur above 23,000 feet.

Short-term acclimatization is usually complete by two weeks. Many riders have a bad day between the second and fifth days at altitude.

TIMING YOUR ARRIVAL AT ALTITUDE

If you are traveling to an important stage race and have the time, arrive three weeks early. You can ride at an easy pace for the first few days, be over the worst altitude effects by one week, train hard the second, and taper slightly the third. If you can't put aside this much time, it may be best to arrive at the last possible moment and hope for the best.

Many races take place over a range of altitudes. If you haven't had the time to acclimatize, it may be better to rest and sleep at lower elevations.

RESTING HEART RATE CHANGES AT ALTITUDE

During travel to altitude, there is a rise in resting heart rate for a week or two, although there may be a short small dip in the middle of the first week. A fall in resting heart rate back to baseline is a measure of acclimatization.

VO_2 MAX AT ALTITUDE

At 5,000 feet, VO_2 max, or the body's maximum ability to use oxygen, is reduced by about 5%. At 6,500 feet, it is reduced by about 7.5%. Thinking about training at Pikes Peak or riding up Mt. Evans in Colorado? There will be a reduction of about 25% in your VO_2 max.

The reduced amount of oxygen means that less work can be performed. Cycling time trial records are often accomplished at altitude because the reduced ability to work is more than compensated for by reduced air resistance. But athletes in sports with less aerodynamic benefit, such as runners, do worse in aerobic events at altitude.

Even when adapted, you cannot sustain the same levels of aerobic work as you can at sea level. For a given workload, your heart rate may be higher. Since you cannot work as hard at altitude, your threshold working heart rate may be lower. For a given speed on the level, your heart rate may be lower.

ACID-BASE BALANCE AT ALTITUDE

At altitude, the acid-base balance in the body changes. This happens because carbon dioxide levels in the blood fall as a result of faster breathing. This changes the blood pH and results in loss of bicarbonate from the kidneys. In this way, the body is less able to buffer lactic acid. However, other mechanisms more than compensate and result, in fact, in decreased lactate levels as described below.

DEHYDRATION, SUNBURN AT ALTITUDE

The air at altitude is usually very dry. Extra fluids may be lost because of increased breathing. Since fluid losses are greater, it's easier to get dehydrated. Sun intensity is also higher. Be sure to drink plenty of fluids, and protect your skin and lips with sunscreens.

Acclimatization—How the Body Adjusts

Adaptations to altitude are long-term and short-term. Long-term adaptations and physiologic changes of altitude living can take months or years. The body adapts to altitude in several ways. Here's how:

INCREASED BREATHING

After first ascending to altitude, breathing may increase as much as 65%. This initial effect is limited. Increased breathing blows off carbon dioxide and increases blood pH, which, in turn, inhibits breathing. This inhibition fades with time, but later, rates may increase again, up to 500% of normal.

INCREASED HEMOGLOBIN IN THE BLOOD

Hemoglobin, the blood protein that carries oxygen, may increase from 15 to 22 grams per 100 milliliters of blood. The hematocrit, the percentage of red blood cells in the blood, may increase from 40–45 to 60–65. This degree of change occurs only in some people at extremely high altitudes. How much extra hemoglobin is made depends on how high one ascends and how long one is exposed to reduced oxygen levels. Generally, increases are more modest. Hemoglobin/hematocrit usually increases about 4% for every 1,000 meters (3,000 feet) of elevation above sea level. The volume of blood is reported to increase in some studies, to decrease in others.

The net effect is this: Studies show that the total circulating hemoglobin may increase, in extreme circumstances, from 50% to 90%. Increases in the 10% to 20% range are more common in athletes who live or train at altitude. The increase results from the naturally produced hormone erythropoetin (EPO). Studies show that EPO levels begin to rise significantly in two hours, and evidence suggests that exposure to an elevation of 8,000 feet for six hours daily will raise hemoglobin levels approximately 10% after two to three weeks. Further increases may occur with more prolonged exposure to higher altitudes.

ETHICS AND SYNTHETIC EPO

Erythropoetin (EPO) is a hormone released by the kidney that stimulates the bone marrow to make red blood cells. This hormone has been produced synthetically since the early 1990s. There is good reason to believe that this substance can help human performance. But, artificially increased numbers of red blood cells may result in thick blood that clots. This has been reported to be responsible for athletes' deaths.

Altitude has a similar effect but may produce some protection against this, and the body has regulatory mechanisms governing the quantities of EPO produced. Athletes may take synthetically produced EPO in quantities higher than those produced in response to altitude. One hears about EPO causing death in athletes;

one doesn't hear about this problem in residents of Mammoth, California; Park City, Utah; or other high-altitude cities.

There's another problem: EPO is a banned substance.

INCREASED DIFFUSING CAPACITY OF THE LUNGS

The lungs exchange gases, taking in oxygen and giving up carbon dioxide. The normal volume of gases exchanged, per minute, increases at altitude. This may be due to either (1) increased pulmonary capillary volume, caused by expanded capillaries and increased surface area, or (2) increased lung volume.

INCREASED VASCULARITY OF TISSUES

The body responds to reduced oxygen by making more blood vessels. Studies have shown that the smallest blood vessels, capillaries, become more concentrated in muscle. This adaptation may take months to years.

INCREASED ABILITY OF CELLS TO USE OXYGEN

Myoglobin, the muscle protein that transports oxygen, increases about 15%. There are increased mitochondria—the energy factories of cells. Some studies have shown an increase in 2,3 DPG, a chemical that helps release oxygen to the tissues. Oxidative enzymes are increased.

DECREASED LACTATE LEVELS WITH EXERTION

Studies show that exposure to high altitude results in decreased lactate levels for a given workload. This could be due to increased levels of myoglobin and hemoglobin, both of which buffer acids, or an increase in certain enzymatic pathways. Altitude exposure decreases bicarbonate—this works against improved buffering.

How Altitude Effects Could Help Cyclists

Increased hemoglobin results in increased aerobic capacity. This improves the aerobic fitness of the athlete. The increased vascularity of tissues and the increased ability of the cells to use oxygen could also help athletes, but these effects take months to develop.

Since cycling balances aerobic and muscular fitness, increased aerobic capacity means that the balance of gear selection shifts to a higher r.p.m. This improves the response to the changing accelerations that characterize cycling events.

How Altitude Effects Could Hurt Cyclists

Less ability to do high-level work may lead to detraining: a loss of muscle mass, a loss of anaerobic power, and a loss of threshold ability. As stated above, altitude may decrease the body's ability to buffer lactic acid because of the loss of bicarbonate. Altitude sickness may lessen the athlete's ability to train.

Many elite athlete teams travel to altitude camps. Although such camps can be good for training, contagious illnesses (such as cold and stomach flu) and the stress of traveling and performing are not good for all athletes. And many athletes are plagued by boredom when they are away from home.

Altitude and Sea-Level Performance—Study Results

There is little doubt that exposure to altitude helps altitude performance. But does it help sea-level performance? Whether altitude camps, where athletes work and sleep, improve sea-level performance is a subject of long-standing controversy.

Of the studies performed to date, about half were uncontrolled: athletes training at altitude did not have a matched group training at sea level. Although the studies are imperfect, about 25% found no difference in sea-level performance, about 40% found worse performance, and about 35% found improved performance. As a whole, the studies found no clear benefit of altitude training for sea-level performance.

Altitude Resting

WHAT WE'RE TALKING ABOUT

There are good physiological reasons why acclimatization to altitude might help sea-level performance. But there are also reasons why it might worsen performance, chief among them the impossibility of intense, high-level workouts at altitude.

Some have reasoned that the best of all worlds would be to train at sea level and rest at altitude. There are at least three approaches:

1. In a geographically convenient location, live at altitude and commute to training workouts at a lower elevation.
2. Live and work out at sea level, but sleep and/or rest in an altitude chamber.
3. Live and work out at sea level, but simulate altitude for sleeping and/or resting by reducing the density of oxygen through the use of nitrogen as substitute gas.

WHAT STUDIES SHOW

Half a dozen studies have specifically addressed living or sleeping high and training low. All studies have shown that living high and training low improves performance.

Conclusion

It's agreed that acclimatization to altitude is helpful for altitude performance. What we've discussed is whether altitude can enhance sea-level performance.

Table 2-14 **Summary of Selected Altitude Studies**

Live/Sleep	Train	Effect on Sea-Level Performance	
Altitude	Altitude	No effect	3 of 12 studies
		Positive effect	4 of 12 studies
		Negative effect	5 of 12 studies
Altitude	Sea level	Positive effect	6 of 6 studies

Traditionally, studies have examined whether altitude training camps are helpful. But there are two other possibilities: the use of altitude (or reduced oxygen) only while training, and the use of altitude (or reduced oxygen) only while resting and/or sleeping. Studies have evaluated the use of altitude for the enhancement of sea-level performance. Some studies have shown a benefit, but just as many have shown a worsening effect or no effect on human performance. There are good physiologic reasons why altitude might benefit human performance; there are also reasons why it might worsen it.

Living and/or sleeping at altitude, while training at sea level, may combine the best of all worlds—the good physiologic effects, without the bad. Every one of six studies reviewed showed a benefit.

Supplemental Oxygen

The use of higher than normal levels of oxygen, either by increasing the concentration of oxygen in the air breathed, or by increasing the atmospheric pressure around the athlete, has been proposed to help athletes.

Pressure Chambers for Resting

Oxygen in the blood exists in two forms: bound to hemoglobin, and dissolved in blood. Since hemoglobin is normally fully saturated (96% to 99%) at rest at sea level, in order to meaningfully increase oxygen delivery to tissues it is necessary to increase dissolved oxygen. It takes considerable pressure to do this effectively. At sea level, about 3% of oxygen delivered to tissues is due to dissolved blood. Doubling atmospheric pressure from 14.7 to 29.4 pounds per square inch (760 to 1,520 millimeters Hg), with normal air (21% oxygen) results in an increase of only about 3% in the amount of oxygen in blood.

Hyperbaria (high pressure, generally at several times normal atmospheric pressure, with 100% oxygen) has important medical uses—for example, in treating diving-related problems, wounds, carbon monoxide poisoning, and some infections.

A commercially available portable chamber has been useful at Mt. Everest. It increases "normal air" air pressure by 3 p.s.i., or about one-fifth of an atmosphere. The 3 p.s.i. change is equivalent to coming down 5,000 to 10,000 feet and is helpful in treating altitude sickness. This chamber is promoted to athletes. But for athletes at sea level, whose blood is already almost fully saturated with oxygen, this represents an almost negligible change in blood oxygenation. The commercial advertising for this product implies that resting in the chamber for a few hours a week will improve recovery. I can't find any way of measuring the recovery promoted, or any scientific studies to support this approach.

Increased Oxygen During Exercise

The idea is that increasing oxygen availability will increase the ability to work when blood would otherwise be desaturated of oxygen. This occurs in some sea-level athletes at high levels of exertion, and in all athletes working at high altitude.

The U.S. Olympic Cycling team experimented with this approach during training for the 1996 Olympics. Interval workloads could be increased about 10%. The coaches also found that the athletes required longer recovery times.

The use of oxygen during competition is impractical. Respiratory rates at high levels of exertion are frequently over 100 liters per minute. Delivering this volume of air requires a stationary athlete. The effects of supplemental oxygen last only a few minutes. Even in the most controlled bicycle racing situation—the track—benefits would be lost by the time the rider began to race.

Conclusion

Supplemental oxygen may allow athletes to increase training intensity. It has little role during actual competition. There's no evidence that it helps recovery.

Part Three

GENERAL PREVENTION AND TREATMENT OF INJURIES

Bicycle Safety

Prevention is the best strategy.

- Keep bicycle equipment safe: well maintained and in mechanically sound working order.
- Acquire the riding skills and techniques to operate a bicycle safely.
- Know how bicycle-car accidents commonly occur. Ride in a safe and defensive manner.
- Use specialized safety equipment.

Safe-Functioning Bicycle Equipment

The essentials of a safe-functioning bicycle are these:

- Proper size and fit
- Functioning brakes and gears
- Tightened fastened parts, including wheels, handlebars, and headset
- Aligned frame and true wheels
- Properly inflated tires
- Freely moving drive train

Safe Riding Skills and Techniques

In order to ride a bicycle safely, one must learn how to

- Ride in a straight line
- Look back while riding
- Signal to motorists
- Brake
- Shift gears
- Deal with obstacles, including railroad tracks and dogs

Safe and Defensive Riding Style

Bicycle-car collisions account for only 10% to 20% of accidents, although they are what worry most cyclists and what cause the most serious accidents. Falls account for about 50% of accidents; bicycle-bicycle collisions, 10% to 20%. Bike-dog incidents and other causes split the remainder.

- Obey the traffic code. The bicycle is treated as a vehicle in most states. Learn the local bicycle laws and regulations.
- You are sharing the road with others. Respect the rights of others, and be tolerant if they trespass on yours.
- Assume that motorists will not see you. They expect and look for other motorists; they often have a "blind eye" for cyclists. Anticipate that a motorist will do something imprudent—for example, pull out in front of you.
- Look ahead of your current position. Don't just look at the roadway beneath you. Anticipate possible problems down the road.
- Ride only one person on a bicycle unless there is more than one seat—a tandem or other special bicycle.
- Ride on the right side of the road, not on the left, and not on the sidewalk.
- Do not ride against traffic on one-way streets.
- Keep your hands on the handlebars. Do not ride no-hands.
- Use lights when riding at night.
- Do not ride through stop signs or red lights.
- Don't hitch rides by holding onto or drafting other vehicles.
- Avoid riding under the influence of drugs, including alcohol.
- Signal turns.
- Ride predictably in a straight line at a steady pace.
- Yield to larger roads.
- Look left, right, and left again before entering roads or intersections.
- Make eye contact with drivers. If you don't think they have seen you, shout politely and loudly, "Watch out!"
- Do not use headphones.
- When riding alongside parked cars, look through rear windows to see drivers, and anticipate that car doors may open.
- Even though you have the right of way, do not insist upon it. Cars have much better protection against accidents than you do; you are more likely to be hurt than the motorist.

Safety Equipment

PROTECTION EQUIPMENT

A helmet is an essential and vital piece of safety equipment. Never ride without one. See "Head Injury," page 233. Gloves protect against common hand scrapes that occur with most falls. They also provide comfort and prevent blistering, jarring, overuse, and hand-nerve injuries.

VISIBILITY EQUIPMENT

Lights are often required at night. Bright clothing is also useful. Vertical or horizontal flags are necessary for recumbents, helpful to touring riders, and used by many commuters.

OTHER EQUIPMENT

Mirrors are considered essential by many riders. Bells help alert others to your presence.

First Aid Kit

Prepare a first aid kit. Keep it in your car. Pack it with you when you travel to races. Replace items with expiratory dates as needed.

Basic First Aid Kit

Antibiotic cream (e.g., polysporin) for road rash—2 ounces
Moleskin/Molefoam
2 Iodine swabs (for cleaning of wounds)
10 Regular Band-Aids
1 Tape—1″ wide
6 Aspirin—5-grain tablets
6 Acetaminophen (non-aspirin pain medicine)
2 Antihistamine (e.g. Benadryl tablets, for allergic reactions/stings)
1 Elastic bandage—3″ wide
1 Triangular bandage (for arm sling)
6 Steri-Strips 1/2″ × 4″ (to use across cuts)
5 Non-stick pads 3″ × 4″ (e.g., Telfa, Adaptic; use over wounds and under gauze; or Bioclusive or Tegaderm dressings)
Five 4″ gauze bandage rolls
4 Safety pins
1 Scissors
1 Forceps (tweezers)
1 First aid book and road rash treatment article

Other convenience items, not strictly speaking for first aid, include the following:

- Antacid, liquid
- Antidiarrhea tablets
- Lip balm
- Eyeglass repair kit
- Tampons/sanitary napkins

More Sophisticated Kit—Group or Medical Personnel

- Antibiotics
- Asthma inhaler
- Clavicle splint
- Extra dressings
- Ice packs
- Iodine scrub brush
- Prescription-strength cortisone cream
- Sleeping pills
- Strong pain pills
- Surgical gloves
- Suture and suture instruments
- Wrist support

Rider Down!

A rider falls in your group ride, and may have a serious injury. What do you do?

1. Prevent Further Injury to Rider and Others

Are there other immediate hazards? Are others hurt? Was a car involved in the accident? Is there a danger of explosion? You must evaluate the overall risks of the scene of the accident before attending to the fallen rider.

Get one or two others to act as traffic control—keeping traffic from running over the rider and preventing further injuries. Get other riders and spectators out of the roadway, except those providing necessary assistance. Establish whether the rider has fallen in a relatively safe location, whether the rider's location presents an immoderate risk to self or others, and whether moving the rider immediately is required.

2. Is the Rider Breathing Well?

If the rider is not breathing, CPR may be necessary. If the rider is having trouble breathing, a significant chest injury may be present.

If the rider is breathing normally and talking or cursing, usually there is no need to do anything for at least several minutes. And it usually takes at least several minutes after a fall for a rider to gather his or her wits and be ready to converse intelligently and answer questions.

3. Is Neck Pain Present?

Does the rider have neck pain? Is there movement in both arms and legs? If the rider has neck pain or cannot move some part of all extremities, the rider may have a serious neck or spinal injury and should not be moved.

If the rider has no neck pain and can move the arms and legs, and wishes to move, fine. Never move a rider against his or her will unless there is a serious risk of further injury (for example, because of being in the middle of a heavy traffic lane).

4. Is Arterial Bleeding Present?

Bright red spurting blood signals arterial bleeding. Apply and maintain direct pressure to stop the bleeding.

Several diseases, including AIDS and hepatitis, can be spread by contact with blood or other body fluids. Wear gloves when blood contact will occur. It is frequently possible to direct the rider to apply and maintain pressure.

5. Can the Rider Sit Up?

After being given a few minutes to catch his or her breath, the rider who is unable to sit up unassisted will probably need an ambulance and a trip to the ER.

6. Call for Help

If the rider will need an ambulance, call 911. If no riders in your group have a cellular phone, look for a nearby roadside emergency telephone, or flag down a motorist or two to make the call. There is a good chance that a passing motorist will have a cellular telephone.

7. Hospital Visit Required?

Are there bone injuries? Can the rider easily move the arms and legs? If not, the rider needs a trip to the hospital. Even though a car may be less expensive, consider that an ambulance is a faster ticket into most ERs and may obviate the need for the individual to sit in a waiting room to register. Consider also that a rider can receive needed care while in the ambulance en route to the ER. If it is uncertain whether a trip to the hospital is required at all, why not err on the side of caution?

8. Family Contacts

Contact or make arrangements to contact family members or close friends of the injured if a hospital trip is needed.

9. Remember the Bike

Try to make arrangements for the rider's bicycle to be safely returned.

Bicycle Position

Overuse injuries in bicycling often result from either improper bicycling position or the lack of sufficient time for adaptation to a new position. Proper bicycle position and sufficient time for adaptation to a new position help prevent many injuries.

Certain general principles apply. There is a "window" of perfectly acceptable bike fit. The final decision regarding position must be made by the individual rider.

Bicycle position is a compromise among many bicycling needs. Optimal position is different for maximizing muscle power, aerobic efficiency, and comfort and for minimizing injury.

Too often, riders are "classically" positioned without regard for their individual variations. Riders with anatomical variants—for example, upper or lower extremity discrepancy, or turned-in or turned-out feet—should be fitted to allow for these differences.

Setup

EQUIPMENT

Bicycle, stationary trainer, bike tools, plumb line, level, tape measure, calipers, assistant.

LEVEL BIKE

Set the bicycle on a trainer. Use blocks of wood to raise the front of the trainer to level the bicycle if necessary. Have the seat in a horizontal position to start.

WARM UP

Pedal moderately for at least 10 minutes before adjusting. Pedal moderately for a few minutes between adjustments.

WHERE TO START

The order in which you perform adjustments is important—some measurements are dependent upon others. The order suggested here works best for most riders.

Frame Sizing

For road bikes, measure the inseam and multiply by 65%. This number is a starting point for the frame size you will need. Find the inseam measurement by standing with back to the wall and a 1-inch book binding snug up against the crotch. Measure the distance from the floor to the top of the binding.

Pedal Fore-Aft

The cleat should be positioned so that the ball of the foot is over the pedal spindle. Sprinters may prefer to back their feet out of the pedals a little more and to be more on their toes.

Seat Height—Paramount in Importance

Seat height selection is a compromise between aerobic efficiency, aerodynamics, power, and injury reduction. Cleat thickness, pedal type, and seat tube angle all influence this measurement. Formulas based upon inseam measurements or other body dimensions can only give approximate results and can only provide starting points.

The general idea is that the higher the saddle, the more power you can generate and the less the aerobic cost. You must not be so far extended that your hips rock or that your spin is restricted when you pedal. Some riders determine position by raising the seat until their heels can just clear the pedals. A seat height that results in 25 to 30 degrees of knee flexion when the pedal is at the bottom of the stroke tends to result in the least injury but is not optimal for cycling power or aerobic efficiency.

The higher your seat, the more likely you are to have pain in the back of your knee, Achilles tendon pain, or buttock ache. Those with limited flexibility are the most likely to have problems.

Further discussion about seat height is found in the chapter "Optimal Seat Height," on page 119.

Seat Position Fore-Aft

Some riders position the seat fore-aft by measuring the distance that a plumb line, hanging from the nose of the saddle, falls behind the bottom bracket. Road riders tend to place the seat an inch or more back. Sprinters and time trialists tend to use a more forward position. Other riders determine their seat position by dropping a plumb line from the front of their knees when the cranks are horizontal. They look for the plumb to fall through the pedal axle. For most standard bicycles, road riders usually have their seats all the way back on the rails, time trialists all the way forward, and crit riders in between.

After you have adjusted the fore-aft position, repeat the determination of your seat height, since adjustment of the saddle fore-aft may change the seat height.

Seat Angle

Most riders ride best when the seat is level. Sprinters, aero time trialists, and women may prefer to have the noses of their saddles point down slightly. Climbers may prefer to have the noses point up slightly.

Pedal Rotation Angle

The cleat should be positioned so that your toes point nearly straight ahead. Some riders prefer their feet pointed slightly in, some slightly out. You may wish to ride a little with your cleats slightly loose, and see where you are most comfortable before the final tightening. Cleat position is not as critical with free-rotation systems. In general, if the outside of your knee hurts, adjust your cleats to point your toes a little more outward. If the inside of your knee hurts, point your toes a little more inward.

Stem Height

The stem may be from one to three inches below the height of your saddle. The lower the stem, the more aerodynamic you'll be. If the stem is too low, you may be uncomfortable, especially in your lower back, or you may lose power.

Stem Extension

Most bikes are sized so that most men end up needing stems 10 to 13 centimeters and most women require stems several centimeters shorter. When you are in the drop position, there should be scant clearance between your elbows and your knees, and your back should be flat. A rule of thumb is that the top of the bars should obscure the front axle when you are looking down with your hands in the drops.

Mountain bikers often prefer a combination of longer top tube and shorter stem for better handling on cross-country trails and downhills.

Handlebar Shape

The shape of the handlebar varies with the type of riding. For general road riding, a long top horizontal section is preferred for climbing comfort. The drop of handlebars is partially determined by the comfort level of your hands in the curve.

Handlebar Width

The handlebar width should be roughly the width of your shoulders.

Handlebar Angle

The handlebars should be angled so that the drops are perpendicular to your seat tube. This means that they are pointed down about 15 degrees.

Brake Levers

The brake levers are most comfortable when they are so positioned that their tips are in line with the bottom of the handlebar drops.

Toe Clips and Straps

Remember those? If you use them, make sure that there is a small clearance between the tip of your shoes and the clip. Make sure the toe straps are at the outside edge of your shoes.

Stretching

Why Stretch?

Stretching may help prevent injuries and strains. Be cautious about stretching when injured. Use stretching primarily to prevent reinjury.

Stretching is effective in increasing flexibility. Joint motion is limited by joint capsules, ligaments, and muscles. These tissues can be successfully elongated with stretching exercises. Some stretching has a merely temporary effect, based on the elastic properties of the tissue stretched. Other effects of stretching can be long-lasting.

Stretching is obviously important in athletic efforts such as gymnastics. Whether or not increased flexibility results in improved performance in bicycling is subject to some debate. Most coaches and bicyclists who stretch believe it is helpful. Hard "scientific" evidence showing this to be the case, however, is lacking.

Guidelines

- A stretch workout can be done in 15 minutes. If you have the time it can easily occupy a half hour.
- Develop a stretching routine, and perform your stretches in the same order. Such a routine helps you perform all your stretches and not miss any.
- Stretch the muscle groups that are the most important for you early in your routine. That way, if you are interrupted and don't finish your stretching, you will have at least stretched what is most important.
- Some joints can be stretched in several directions. Develop your routine so as to stretch these complementary motions in sequence. For example, after bending your back as in Figure 3-16, page 157, arch it as in Figures 3-17 and 3-18.
- Stretch slowly and gradually. Avoid bouncing or ballistic motions. There is a basic neurologic reflex called the stretch reflex. When a muscle is suddenly stretched, the reflex contracts, or shortens, the muscle. If you stretch slowly, the reflex is not activated. Fast stretching is usually counterproductive.
- Stretch to tightness, but not to the point of pain.
- Hold stretches for at least 20 seconds and up to 60 seconds.
- Stretching is more effective when the muscles are warm, not cold. Avoid stretching first thing in the morning when you are otherwise stiff. If your routine provides the time to stretch in the morning, first ride your

stationary trainer easily for 10 minutes, or do some other general exercise. Stretching is probably more helpful after a bicycle ride than before one.

Put Your Mind in Your Muscle

Concentrate on how the muscles being stretched feel during the stretch. This will aid in ensuring proper tension and help you to maximize gains, utilize proper form, and prevent stretching injury.

If you pay more attention to the range of motion than to how the muscle feels, the tendency will be for you to "cheat" yourself. For example, when performing the hamstring stretch (Figure 3-12, page 155), if you focus on placing your head to your knee, the tendency will be to bend the back and flex the neck forward in an effort to "help" get the head to the knee. But the hamstrings may not be properly stretched!

A more productive form would be to isolate the stretch on the target muscles—the hamstrings—by keeping the back and the neck straight. Even though there may now be many inches between your head and knee, the hamstrings will receive a more productive stretch.

Definitions

Flexion: bending in of a body part. Generally, movement of a joint that results in the two parts of it coming closer together.
Extension: straightening out of a body part. To move a joint to place the two parts of it farther apart.
Abduction: movement away from the midline of the body.
Adduction: movement toward the midline of the body.

Where illustrations in Figures 3-1 through 3-24 show one side of the body, the right-side stretch is shown. Stretch both sides!

Figure 3-1

Trunk range of motion. Perform five times clockwise, then five times counterclockwise.

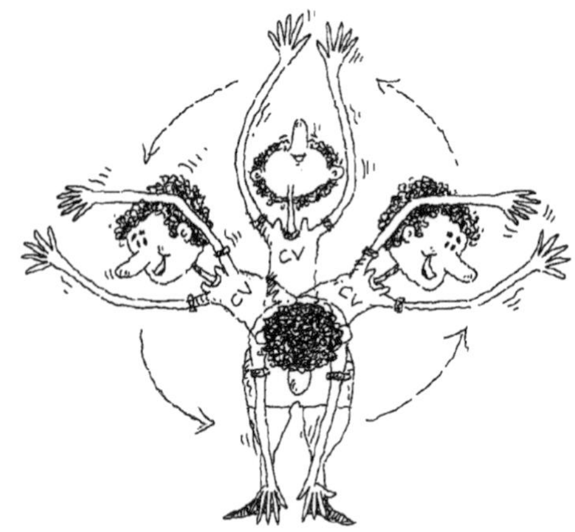

Figure 3-2

Neck stretch. Illustration shows side-to-side. Also perform up and down. Rotation of the head in circles is controversial.

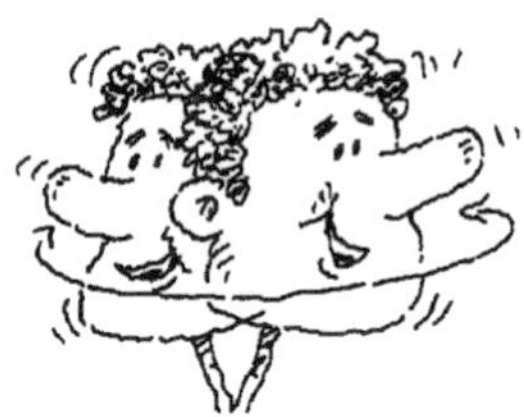

Figure 3-3

Calf stretch. Perform with straight knee to stretch gastrocnemius and Achilles tendon. Keep foot flat. Also stretches sole of foot.

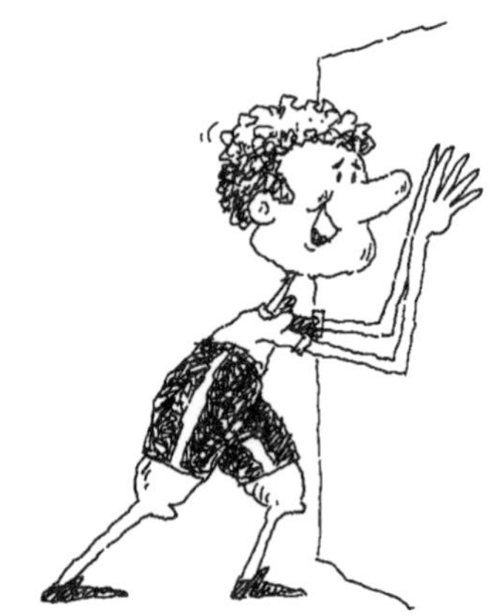

Figure 3-4

Calf stretch. Perform with bent knee to stretch the soleus and the Achilles tendon. Keep the foot flat. Also stretches sole of foot.

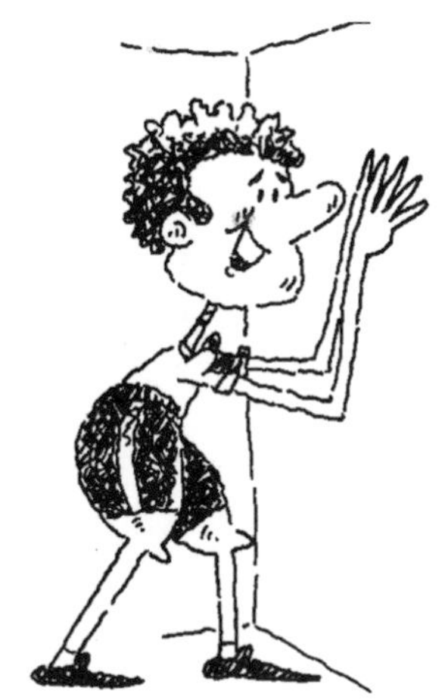

Figure 3-5

Quad stretch. Grab ankle or foot and pull back to buttocks, flexing knee. Then extend hip, pulling knee back, to complete stretch.

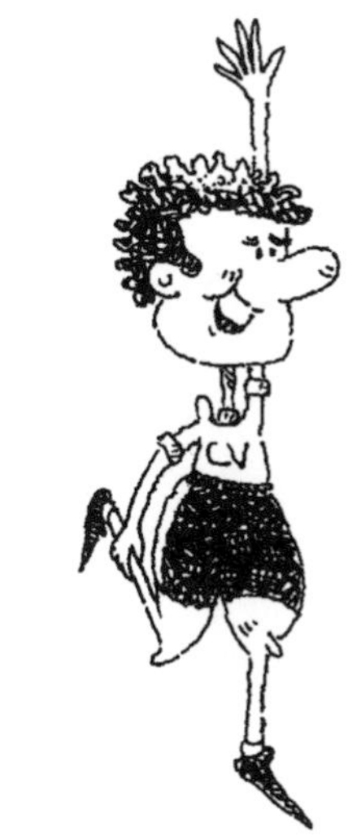

Figure 3-6

Hip flexors, groin stretch. Move one leg forward until knee of forward leg is directly over ankle, other knee resting on floor. Lower the front of your hip downward.

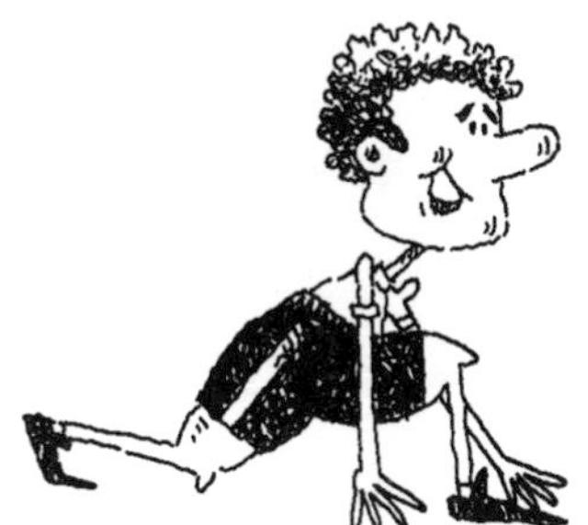

Figure 3-7

Adductor stretch. Stand with legs apart. Bend one knee. Pivot toward bent knee to stretch adductors of straight leg.

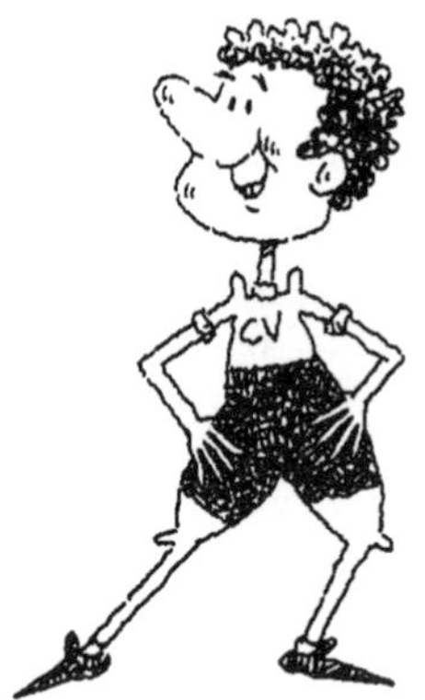

Figure 3-8

Abductor, iliotibial band stretch. Cross ankles. Using wall for support, press inside leg against outside leg to stretch abductors and iliotibial band of outside leg.

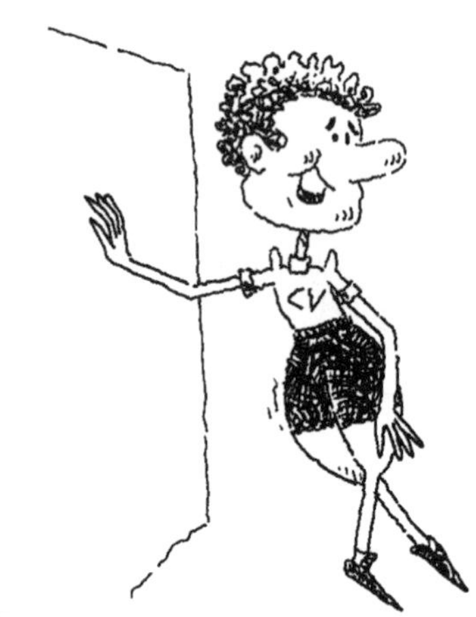

Figure 3-9

Iliotibial band stretch. Lie on side, leg to be stretched on top. Slightly bend other leg. Hold foot; bring knee forward. Rotate knee in a circle up, round, and down. When knee is held down by groin muscles, ITB stretch occurs.

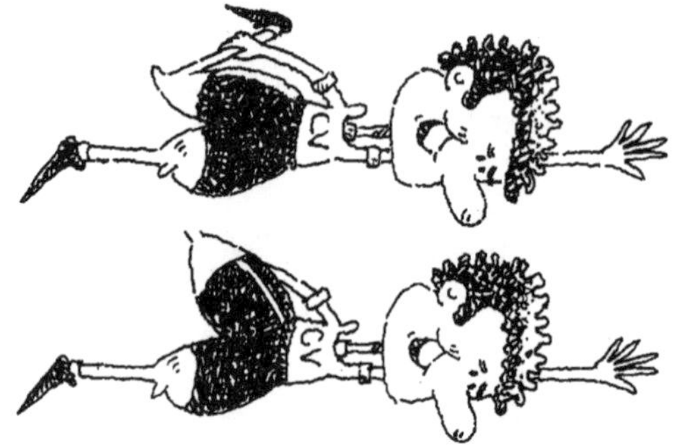

Figure 3-10
Groin, hip adductor stretch. Sit against the wall, soles of feet together. Lean forward, bending from hips, not shoulders. Use your elbows to help stretch your knees outward.

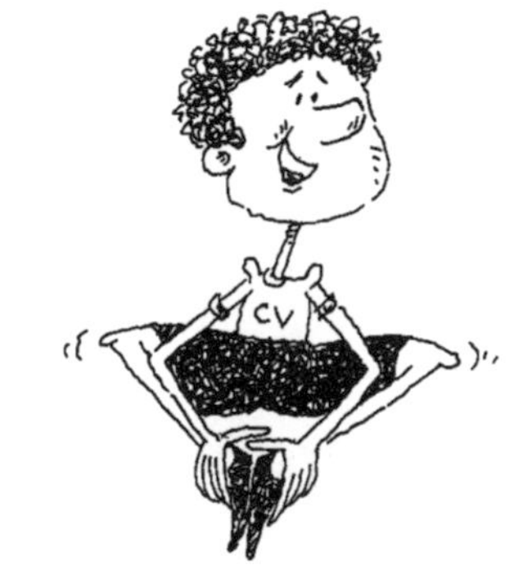

Figure 3-11

Hip adductor, hamstring stretch. Feet spread apart, perhaps against a wall. Bend forward. If you perform face to face with a partner, hold each other's hands, gently pull forward. Or pull on rope or towel fastened to object in front of you.

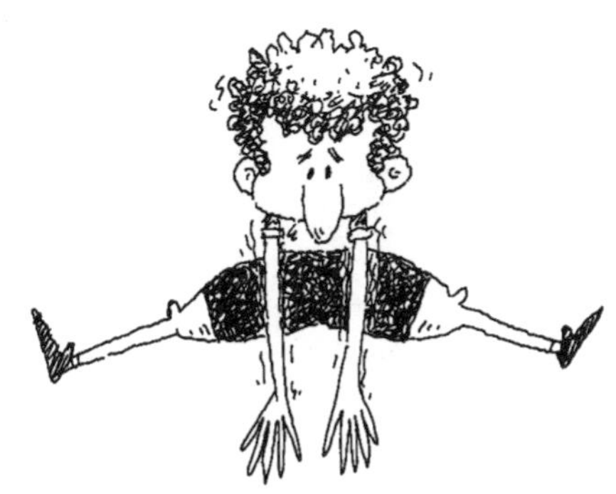

Figure 3-12

Hamstring stretch. Straighten right leg. Set sole of left foot in toward crotch. Hold onto leg, ankle, or foot as able. Lean forward from hips; keep back straight.

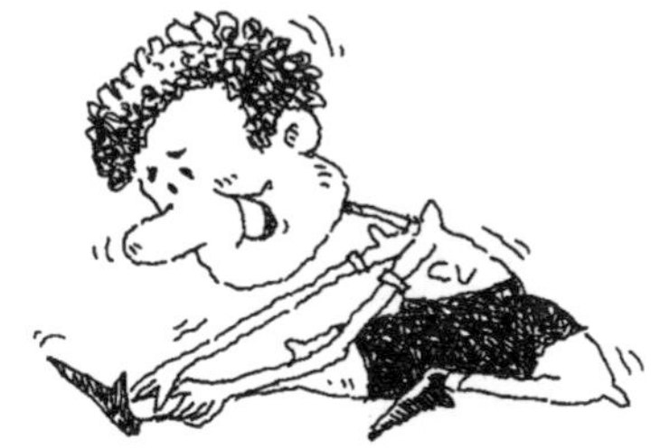

Figure 3-13

Hamstring stretch. Bend forward; hold legs, ankles, or feet as able. Bend from hips, keep back straight, pull gently.

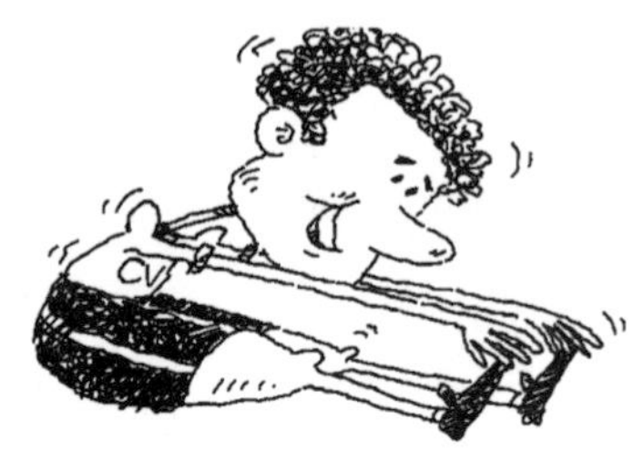

Figure 3-14

Piriformis stretch. Lie down; flatten back. Bend right knee; cross leg over left leg. Anchor right foot against left knee. Use hand to pull right knee over left leg and toward floor. Keep shoulders flat.

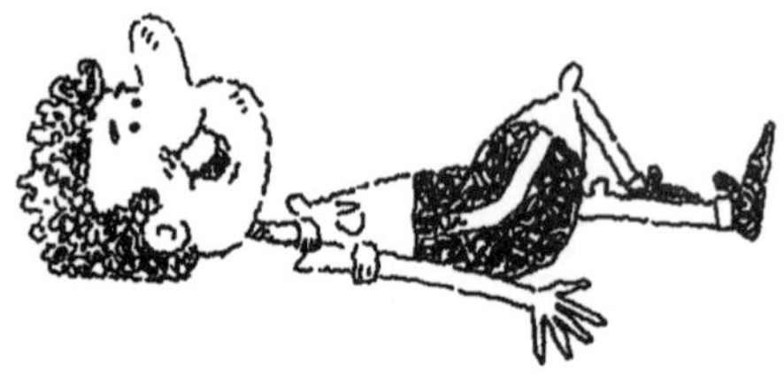

Figure 3-15

Back rotation stretch. Right leg straight. Put left foot outside of right knee, left knee bent. Bend left elbow and rest on inside of left knee. With right hand resting behind, turn head to look over right shoulder and rotate body toward right hand and arm. Can also be performed with right elbow on outside of left knee, turning in the other direction. This may also stretch the left buttock.

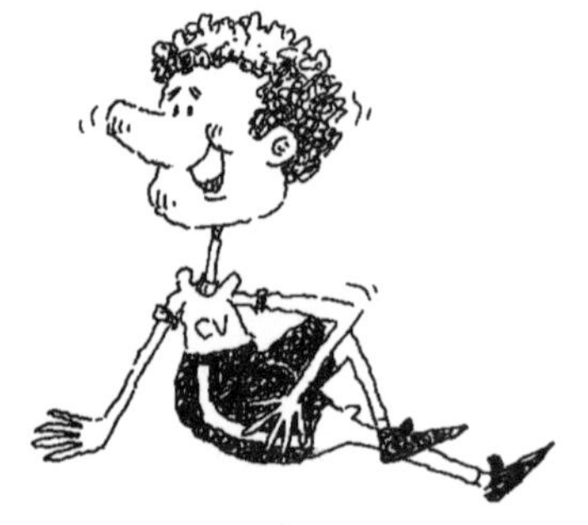

Figure 3-16

Back flexion stretch. Also flexion stretch of the neck. It may take a while to be able to place your feet on the floor behind you.

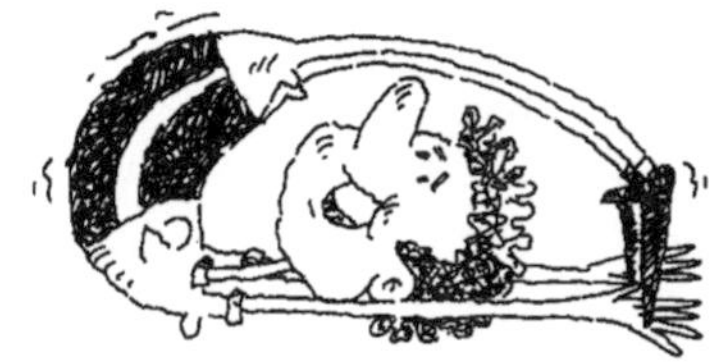

Figure 3-17

Back extension stretch. Lie face down. Push up with arms while arching back and looking up toward the ceiling. Back should become curved in a smooth fluid motion.

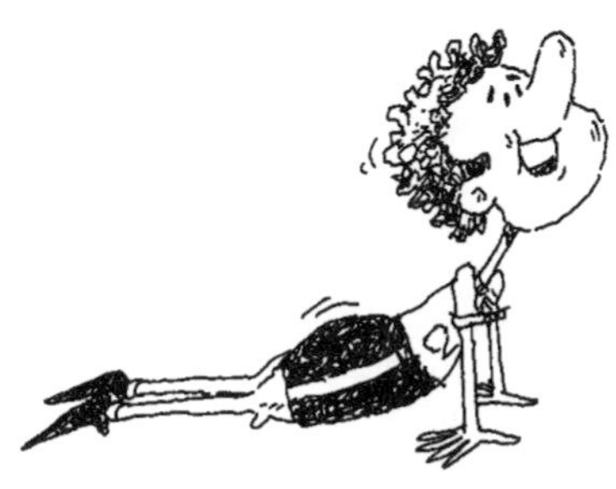

Figure 3-18

Back extension stretch. Also extension stretch of neck and flexion stretch of the quadriceps. Lie prone; hold ankles. Pull ankles toward buttocks; extend torso and neck.

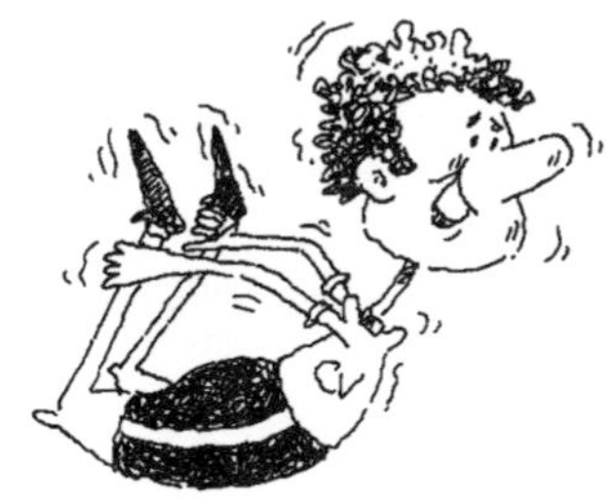

Figure 3-19

Shoulders, arms, upper back stretch. Place hands shoulder width apart on wall. Let upper body droop down. Have knees slightly bent, hips over knees. Knees bent a little more or hands at another height will give a slightly different stretch.

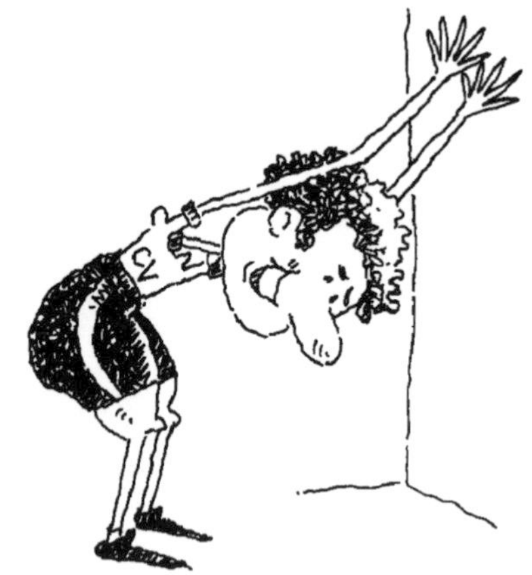

Figure 3-20

Triceps, lateral upper back stretch. Arms overhead, hold elbow of one arm with other hand. Gently pull elbow behind head as you bend hips to side.

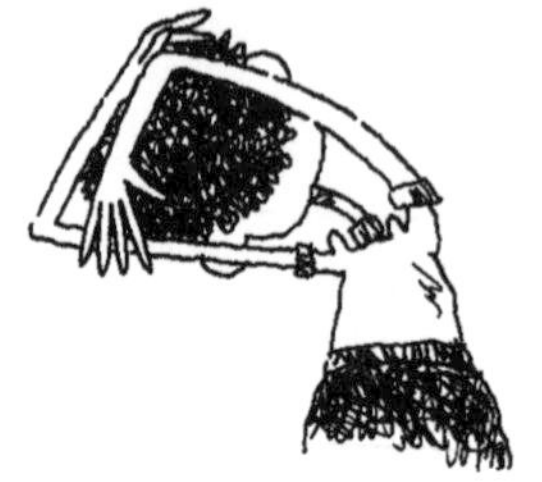

Figure 3-21

Arm, shoulder, upper back stretch. Interlace fingers above head. Face palms upward. Push arms slightly back and up.

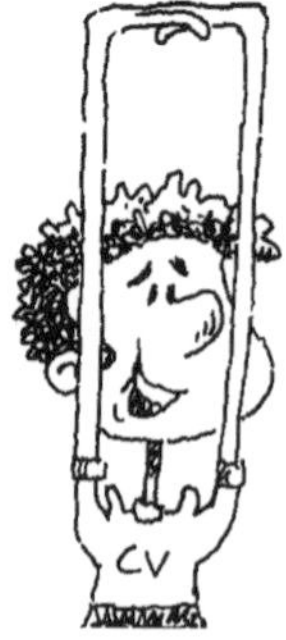

Figure 3-22

Shoulder, arm stretch. Interlace fingers behind back. Turn elbows inward while straightening arms.

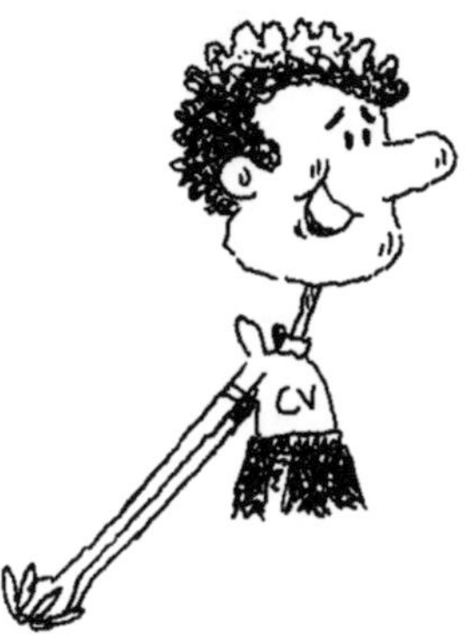

Figure 3-23

Tennis elbow—lateral epicondylitis stretch. The position of maximal stretch of wrist extensors is with elbow extended, forearm turned in, wrist flexed.

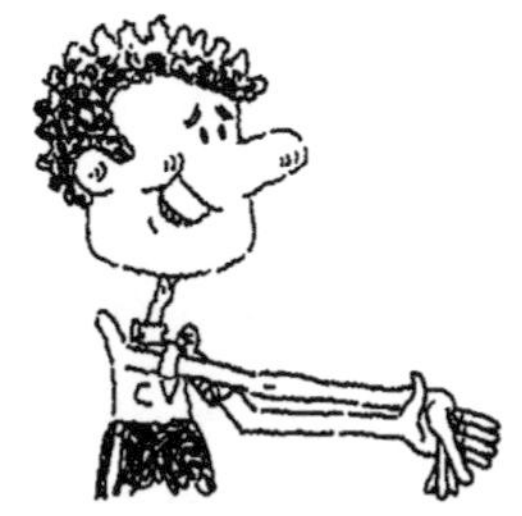

Figure 3-24

Reverse tennis elbow— medial epicondylitis stretch. The position of maximal stretch of wrist flexors is with elbow extended, forearm turned out, wrist back flexed.

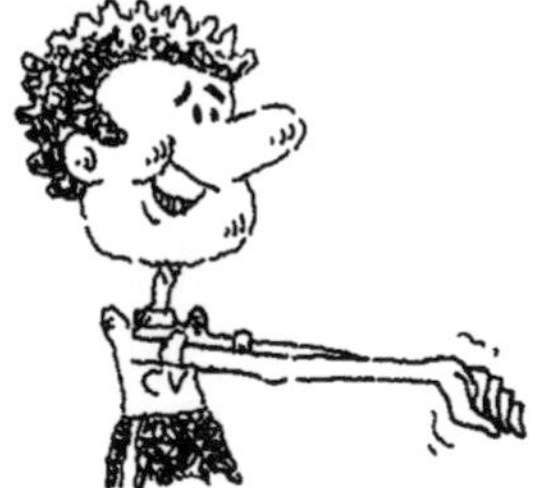

Banned Substances

Assume It's Banned

If you compete, you should assume that anything you ingest except "real food" is banned unless you know otherwise. Banned substances may vary in different countries. If you need to know about a substance, call the United States Olympic Committee drug hotline at 800-233-0393.

Banned substances do not necessarily mean that the drugs are bad, dangerous, or against civil or criminal laws. It means that they are banned from competition. This may be because they may provide an unfair advantage to the athlete, may be dangerous in the quantities used by athletes, may be ethically questionable, or are illegal.

Commonly Used Substances Are Often Banned

Over-the-counter decongestants, used for colds and the flu, are banned. Nose sprays are banned. Most asthma medicines are banned. Many high blood pressure medicines are banned. Many pain pills are banned. Many teas and herbal remedies contain banned substances.

Prohibited substances include the following:

- Stimulants, including amphetamines, caffeine, cocaine, ephedrine, isoproteranol, metaproteranol, phenylpropramine, salbutamol, terbutaline
- Narcotics, including codeine dihydrocodeine, hydrocodeine, methadone, morphine, pentazocine
- Diuretics, including furosemide, hydrochlorthiazide
- Peptide hormones, including ACTH, erythropoetin, growth hormone
- Anabolic steroids, including nandrolone, oxandrolone, stanozol, testosterone
- Masking agents, including probenecid

Exceptions

Some substances—for example, asthma inhalers—needed for medical conditions can be used with prior notification to governing sports bodies. In the U.S., have your physician notify the USOC and USA Cycling. Some substances—for example, caffeine—are acceptable in limited quantities. Assume that any substance is banned unless you know otherwise.

NSAIDs: Non-Steroidal Anti-Inflammatory Drugs

What We're Talking About

Medicines that combat inflammation. These medicines also help reduce pain. A few are available over the counter, such as aspirin, ibuprofen (Advil), and naproxen (Aleve). The rest are obtainable by prescription only.

Many medical problems are due to inflammation, which is the body's healing reaction to injury or infection. The inflammatory response includes warmth, redness, swelling, and local discomfort. Sometimes the body fights too hard, and excessive inflammation leads to needless pain, discomfort, or disability.

Non-steroidal anti-inflammatory drugs are a mainstay of medical treatment. Not only do they provide temporary relief, they may reduce the vicious circle of injury, inflammation, swelling and persistent injury. When overuse injury is the problem, they are not a substitute for correct bicycle fit and/or the development of true physical adaptation.

Problems with NSAIDs

A common problem with this class of medicines is that they upset the gastrointestinal (GI) tract. I've listed the relative amounts of GI upset caused by these medicines in Table 3-1. On a scale of 1 to 4, 1 is minimal; 4 is a lot.

Aspirin and ibuprofen last for only a few hours and so often require many daily doses to be helpful. Several medicines in the group need to be taken only once or twice a day. Sometimes one works well where the others do not. Dosing frequency is also listed in the table.

If these medicines cause gastrointestinal problems or you need them for more than a couple of weeks, consult your physician.

Table 3-1 **NSAIDs — Common Agents, Dose, and Side Effects**

Class and Agent	Doses a Day*	GI Side Effects
Fenamates		
Meclofenamate sodium (Meclomen)	4	3
Mefenamic acid (Ponstel)	4	1
Indoles		
Indomethacin (Indocin)	2 – 3	4
Indomethacin (Indocin SR)	1	4
Sulindac (Clinoril)	2	1
Tolmetin sodium (Tolectin)	3 – 4	3
Napthykanone		
Nabumetone (Relafen)	2	2
Oxicam		
Piroxicam (Feldene)	1	3
Phenylacetic acid		
Diclofenac sodium (Voltaren)	4	2
Proprionic acids		
Fenoprofen calcium (Nalfon)	3 – 4	2
Flubiprofen (Ansaid)	3 – 4	2
Ibuprofen (Advil, Motrin)	3 – 4	2
Ketoprofen (Orudis)	3 – 4	2
Naproxen (Naprosyn)	2	2
Naproxen sodium (Naprelan, Aleve, Anaprox)	1 – 2	2
Oxaprosin (Daypro)	1	1
Pyranocarboxylic acid		
Etodolac (Lodine)	3	1
Pyrazoles		
Phenylbutazone (Azoid, Butazolidin)	4	4
Pyrrolopyrrole		
Ketorolac tromethamine (Toradol)	4	3
Salicylates		
Acetylsalicylic acid (Aspirin)	4	4
Diflunisal (Dolobid)	2	1

* Doses range from 1 to 4 daily. GI upset ranges from 1-minimal to 4-most.

Aspirin May Help

Aspirin Is Inexpensive

Simple aspirin is as strong as most NSAIDs, is much less expensive, and requires no prescription. Unless you have a special problem, the cheapest brand of aspirin is probably the one you should buy. Normally you can get 200 5-grain (325-milligram) aspirin tablets for a couple of dollars. Brand-name aspirin does not work better for most people—it only costs more. "Extra-strength" aspirin is just a bigger dose. Three regular aspirins are virtually the same as two extra-strength tablets.

How to Take Aspirin

Side effects are minimized by taking aspirin with food. There are several ways to take aspirin or other NSAIDs. A dose may be taken when you hurt; you can take a dose in anticipation of inflammation; you may dose regularly to try to cure a long-standing problem.

AS-NEEDED DOSING

You take the medicine when you hurt. If you ride with tendonitis and get sore after a ride, three regular aspirins may help a lot.

ANTICIPATORY DOSING

Alternatively, if you know that after going for a ride you are going to hurt, you might take a few aspirin before your ride to prevent post-ride pain and inflammation.

REGULAR DOSING

Or, if tendonitis has been a problem for you for the last couple of weeks, regularly taking two or three aspirins four times a day (with each meal and at bedtime) may help alleviate your problem.

Correct Dose

The dose of aspirin for inflammation is eight to twelve tablets a day. For regular dosing, the right amount is just less than that which causes ringing in your ears. If you get a ringing in your ears, you should cut back your daily dose by one or two tablets.

Side Effects

If you experience stomach pain or discomfort, you may need to stop aspirin as therapy. If aspirin were a new drug marketed today, it might be available only by prescription.

Aspirin Helps Pain and Inflammation

Remember, NSAIDs help both pain and inflammation. You may want to try aspirin not only for your discomfort but also for inflammation. Reducing inflammation may help you get better faster.

Not Acetaminophen

Acetaminophen (Tylenol, Panadol, Anacin3) is a non-aspirin product that is helpful for pain and fever in much the same way that aspirin is. It does not work against inflammation and may not be the right type of medicine for inflammatory conditions.

Physical Therapy

Physical therapy provides a variety of healing methods for acute and chronic conditions that may result from overuse, degeneration, injury, or surgery. The use of these methods is not restricted to physical therapists. Physicians, athletic trainers, osteopaths, and chiropractors may all have education and experience in using all or some of these methods. Physical therapy involves not only the treatment itself but the education and instruction of patients. It often provides important psychological support for patients.

It may consist of the following types of programs for the following purposes:

Range of Motion Exercises

Increase the range of motion of joints.

PASSIVE RANGE OF MOTION

Joint motion performed without muscle force—either by the patient or by another person. These exercises are sometimes performed with the assistance of gravity or traction as the moving force.

ACTIVE RANGE OF MOTION

Joint motion performed with muscular force. The patient actively uses muscular force to increase range of motion.

Stretching

Increases the length of ligaments or tendons.

Stretching is helpful in preventing and treating overuse injuries. Many overuse injuries are the result of too much stress or tension on a tendon. Stretching the muscles and tendons allows them to absorb more strain without discomfort. Remember, be cautious about stretching when you are injured. Use stretching primarily to prevent re-injury.

Stretching is discussed more on page 150. For some specific overuse injuries, specific stretches are helpful. These are discussed in the overuse injury sections.

Strengthening Programs

Strengthen specific muscles. Strengthening exercises may help to rehabilitate or cure many problems. Be cautious about strength training when you are injured. Use strength training primarily to prevent re-injury.

It is important to understand what the exercise is meant to accomplish and to perform it correctly. For example, leg extensions performed only for the last 20 degrees of extension—so-called short-arc or terminal-extension exercises—help many knee problems. Full-extension exercises worsen many knee problems.

Massage

Provides pain relief and helps muscular relaxation. There is little understanding about how this works. Research has shown that the effectiveness of massage is *not* due to increasing blood flow, improving oxygenation of tissues, or reducing lactic acid levels.

Whirlpool Bath

Provides a massage-type effect. A whirlpool bath is also helpful for the gentle removal of scabs or scablike material from abrasions, burns, or other wounds.

Cold

Prevents local swelling or provides pain relief. It decreases the local circulation. Cold is generally applied intermittently for the first 48 hours after an injury or while swelling is present.

Cold is discussed in greater detail under "Ice" in the "R.I.C.E." chapter beginning on page 167.

Heat

Increases the local circulation and is thought to speed the healing process. It is generally applied after injuries, when swelling has gone down. Heat may be local and applied directly by heating pads, hot-water bottles, or hot baths. It may be local and applied indirectly, as with infrared light. Heat may be deep, such as that provided by diathermy and ultrasound.

If you use heat on your own, use it for no more than 20 minutes at a time every two hours. Be cautious about avoiding burns—I see them frequently from heating pads. Heat should not cause significant pain or redness when applied. Do not use heat or cold on areas of the skin that are numb or that suffer from decreased circulation. It is easy to burn or freeze skin that does not sense temperature properly.

Ultrasound

Sound waves penetrate the tissues to cause local heat. They may also provide benefit by vibrating the tissues, but this is uncertain.

Electrotherapy

Electrical currents applied to the skin may help chronic pain. A common electrotherapy device is the Transcutaneous Electrical Nerve Stimulation (TENS) unit.

Manipulation

Unpopular with the established medical profession because of its association with chiropractic medicine. Studies support its effectiveness for certain specific problems, including back pain.

R.I.C.E.—Rest, Ice, Compression, Elevation

The classic initial treatment of injuries comprises these four parts.

Rest

Rest helps almost all injuries. The degree of rest needed depends on the injury.

For many overuse injuries, modified rest is all that is necessary—a reduction in mileage, a lessening of hill work or of big-gear riding. A minimal ankle twist may require only caution for a day or two to avoid re-injury. A mild ankle sprain may require avoidance of sports for a couple of days.

A severe ankle sprain may require casting—really just a method of enforcing rest for a part of the body. Sometimes, as in the case of a broken bone, complete rest may be required. Partial casts and splints represent less extreme forms of enforced rest.

In general, if activity makes your healing injury more painful, you should avoid the activity.

Ice

The application of local cold reduces injury-induced pain, inflammation, and swelling. The body reacts to injury by "bringing in fighter forces" to heal the injury. A relatively excessive reaction of the body, with excessive local swelling, may cause further pain and disability. Ice can help reduce this.

Apply ice for no more than 15 minutes at a time every hour.

Ice directly applied to the skin can cause skin freezing and damage. Wrap ice in a cloth to prevent direct contact with the skin.

Ice is the "code word" in the R.I.C.E. formula, but is not necessarily used. My preferred cold substance is a package of frozen vegetables. Frozen peas in a bag, for example, conform easily to the surface of the damaged body part and can be used repeatedly. But don't eat those peas after several freeze-thaw cycles!

Compression

Compressing the injured area prevents fluid from entering, reduces swelling, and also provides a modest form of enforced rest.

Avoid compressing so tightly that the circulation is impaired. Compression applied closer to the heart should be less strong than that applied further away. Numbness, tingling, or pale or bluish skin may result from compression that is too tight.

Compression applied before swelling has formed is usually better than that applied after swelling is already present.

Many different products for compression use are on the market. In an ankle injury, for example, an Ace wrap provides modest compression but not much support. Specialty products, such as an ankle Aircast support, provide significantly more effective compression and support.

Elevation

Raising the injured part to the level of the heart reduces local swelling. For example, injuries to the arm are often elevated with a sling. Leg injuries are elevated by sitting and supporting the leg on, for example, another chair.

Other Treatment Options

Orthotics

These shoe inserts help support the foot and direct weight and energy forces. Orthotics may provide support, cant (angle) the foot, or provide a space or shim to help correct a small leg length discrepancy. They are used for a variety of foot, ankle, knee, hip, back, and other biomechanical problems. Cycling orthotics are longer than running orthotics—they should support the metatarsal heads.

Orthotics may be modest over-the-counter products used interchangeably by different individuals and different sports, or sport-specific custom products costing hundreds of dollars.

They may help those in whom anatomic variation is otherwise difficult to correct by adjustment of the bicycle. Orthotics may be helpful in realigning the structures of the leg. They tend to be most useful for problems closer to the foot and less useful for such problems as back and neck ache.

WHO'S MOST LIKELY TO NEED AN ORTHOTIC?

Those who walk with an abnormal pressure pattern are most likely to be helped with orthotics. If you have chronic foot, knee, hip, or leg pain or problems, and your patterns are abnormal, it's possible an orthotic may help.

Figure 3-25

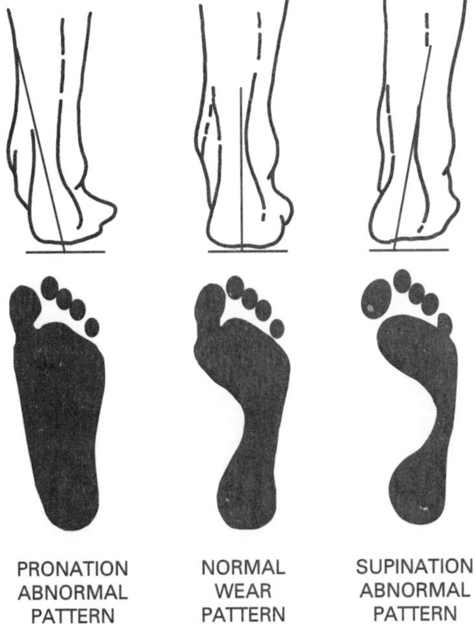

Foot patterns

If your pattern is abnormal and you have no problems, there is no reason to get orthotics. For those who have needed orthotics, studies have shown no difference in power when they cycle with orthotics. Orthotics may help pain or other medical problems but do not otherwise improve performance.

Shims

Leg length discrepancy is usually corrected by a shim placed between the cleat and the shoe. Approximately half the discrepancy is corrected, and the bicycle is adjusted to fit the longer leg. See "Leg-Length Discrepancy," starting on page 209.

Muscle Relaxants

A group of popular medicines. Some pharmacologists dispute their specificity. My personal feeling is that they relax the brain as much as the muscles. Most people have a natural tendency toward depression when injured, and muscle relaxants, I believe, often increase an individual's depression. I do not think they usually have significant value in the treatment of injuries, and hardly ever use them.

Pain Medicine

May be needed for sudden injuries. A combination pill containing Tylenol and codeine is the most widely prescribed pain medicine. This is stronger than over-the-counter medicine.

Codeine is a narcotic. Use what you need for pain control, but don't use more than you need. If aspirin, Advil (ibuprofen) or Tylenol (acetaminophen) is sufficient, there is no need to suffer the narcotic side effects of constipation and mental dullness.

If NSAIDs (anti-inflammatories) are used for inflammation as well as pain control, you may wish to continue their use even after the pain has diminished.

Cortisone

A natural body hormone, cortisone products have also been synthesized as drugs with massive anti-inflammatory potencies. They are available as oral, topical, and injectable medications.

Local injections allow direct placement at the inflamed structure. This is a powerful method of relieving inflammation but has some serious side effects. For example, injected cortisone can cause weakness and rupture of a tendon. For this reason, it is inappropriate for problems with the Achilles and patellar tendons.

Surgery

This is the most invasive tool for solving problems. Sometimes it is the first choice in helping a broken bone or other serious injury. For overuse injuries, surgery is most often a last resort.

Ride or Rest?

What We're Talking About

Your knee aches. Your back is sore. You've got tendonitis in your ankle. Should you take a few days or weeks off the bike? Or is it okay to ride?

Most of the time, we're talking about pains or problems where there isn't a whole lot to see. X rays of that sore knee won't show a break. Examining the knee doesn't show fluid or redness or other problems. It's all a question of how it feels.

What to Do

These types of problems are challenging for riders and their physicians. Often there is no right answer, but here are some guidelines to help.

- If the problem is not bicycling-related overuse—for example, back ache due to lifting—and you've turned the corner and are improving, it's probably okay to ride.
- If there is swelling or other objective signs, rest is wise.
- If the problem is worse after riding, rest is wise.
- If riding won't change fitness—the ride will be of low volume or intensity—why not rest?

Overriding

Sometimes riders become obsessed with riding and putting on the miles. Some will ride even when pain, discomfort, or exhaustion persists. Taking some days off will be beneficial in the long run. Rest and days off the bike are just as important as other aspects of riding.

Sun Care

There is no such thing as a healthy tan.

What We're Talking About

Bicycle riders are exposed to sun, the damaging effects of which are both medical and cosmetic. Medical problems include sun-induced skin cancer and precancerous changes. Cosmetic changes include wrinkling and freckling. The sun's harmful ultraviolet rays may be present even on hazy or cloudy days. Tanning booths, sunlamps, and reflecting beds also increase sun damage.

Prevention

Always wear sunscreen on all sun-exposed areas. It takes more than 1 ounce to protect your body from head to toe. The nose and ears are common skin cancer sites. Use sunscreen, or lip balms containing sunscreen, on your lips.

Sunscreens are rated by their ability to filter the harmful rays of the sun. Skin protective factors (SPFs) indicate the degree of this protection. Higher numbers are better and also more expensive. Look for SPFs of at least 15. Lower numbers do not protect you enough.

Sunscreens are more effective if applied at least 15 minutes before sun exposure starts. If you are driving to ride or race, put your sunscreen on at home, where you can wash your hands thoroughly, so that you don't accidentally rub your eyes and irritate them with sunscreen from your fingers. Don't stay in the sun longer than you otherwise would simply because you have applied sunscreen.

Many specially designed sun-protective clothing articles are now available. Some helmets come with built-in sun visors. Cycling caps with brims, worn under helmets without visors, can help provide protection. Although clothing can be the best sunscreen, loosely woven fabrics may allow the sun's rays through.

"Chemical-free" sunscreens may be of value to those with sensitive skin. Sunscreen with cream or lotion may help those with dry skin. Sunscreen gels, which dry without an oily film, are useful for people with oily skin.

Road rash is likely to burn easily and to leave permanent skin discoloration. Cover it or use sunscreen. Some cosmetics and oral medications can cause reactions when the skin is exposed to the sun.

Other Climate Effects

Additional information concerning environmental effects is found in the "Travel and Climate Problems" chapter on page 124.

Bites, Stings, Infectious Diseases

What We're Talking About

Mosquito bites, bee stings, and wasp stings; tick bites and the danger of Lyme disease; rodent droppings and the danger of Hantavirus; contaminated water and Giardia organisms.

Prevention

A complete description of these problems will not be attempted. Know your local area and its dangers. Avoid infested areas, use insect repellent, do not handle droppings, and do not drink out of streams.

Part Four

MEDICAL PROBLEMS

Classification of Bicycling Medical Problems

Overuse Injuries

Overuse injuries are chronic, uncontrolled, overload, microtraumatic events.

CAUSES

Adaptation

Overuse injuries occur over a period of time when forces applied to a structure are increased faster than the structure can adapt, or exceed its limits of adaptation. Too much too soon is often the cause of problems. Too many miles, or mileage that is too intense, especially on hills and with the use of big gears, often causes overuse injury. Less commonly, excessive spinning may cause problems.

Bicycle Fit

If a rider's fit or position is not optimal, it may contribute to overuse injuries.

Off-the-Bike Activities

Other athletic activities may help or hinder recovery. Weight lifting, running, jumping sports, and racket sports may also cause or contribute to bicycle-related overuse problems.

Weight training has many benefits; it is also taxing on the body. For example, many exercises that specifically strengthen the quadriceps—perhaps the most important bicycling muscle—also place big loads on the kneecap where it glides over the thigh bone. Full squats, leg extensions, and lunges are particularly grueling for knee structures. In the presence of knee pain, some weight training may need to be curtailed.

Running is also stressful on the knee. Running up and especially down hills places tremendous pressures on the knee. Running on inclines, such as along the beach or on the side of a canted road, places stresses on the inside and outside of the knees. In the presence of knee pain, running may need to be stopped.

Anatomy

A person's individual body type and construction may be a contributing factor. For example, some anatomy or body types predispose to certain overuse knee injuries.

- A wide pelvis places the knees farther apart and stresses the outside, or lateral, structures of the knee.
- The shin bone, or tibia, is twisted internally as a normal human variant in many people. This twist results in a tendency for the feet to turn inward. Trying to ride with toes pointed straight ahead may cause discomfort on the inside (medial) aspect of the knee.
- Unbalanced muscles or other anatomical variants may lead to abnormal tracking of the knee cap.
- Leg-length discrepancy is not usually associated with problems in general or recreational riders unless the difference between the legs exceeds 6 millimeters (1/4 inch). However, long-distance riders or racers may experience leg-length discrepancy–related problems with as little as 3 millimeters (1/8 inch) of difference.
- Excessive foot pronation is associated with medial (inside aspect of the) knee pain.

Riders with anatomical variants may require non-standard configurations of their equipment—for example, in the case of leg-length discrepancy, asymmetrically positioned cleats.

GRADING OVERUSE INJURIES

Overuse injuries can be graded according to pain persistence:

Grade 1: Pain only after activity
Grade 2: Pain starts during activity
Grade 3: Pain still persists the next day
Grade 4: Constant pain

PREVENTING OVERUSE INJURIES

General principles apply to overuse injuries in all sports. Allow the body sufficient time to adapt. Increase activity gradually, and allow periods of rest and adaptation—for example, by alternating heavy and light workouts. A warmup and cooldown, and stretching before and after, may help. In bicycling, warmup, cooldown, and stretching are more important for track racers than for road riders.

OVERUSE TREATMENT PRINCIPLES

The following treatment methods, as well as stretching and strengthening programs, are discussed in more detail in Part Three, beginning on page 139.

1. *Adjust activity to allow healing.* Adjusted activity may be partial to complete rest.
2. *Reduce inflammation.* Ice, oral non-steroidal anti-inflammatory drugs (NSAIDs), cortisone injections, and physical therapy, including ultrasound, electrical stimulation, and contrast baths, are common ways to reduce inflammation.
3. *Correct biomechanical stress or external factors.* In bicycling, assure correct or modified bicycle fit and cleat placement. Bicycle fit must be individualized to the injured rider—it may not be the "correct" position for the average uninjured rider. Some medical problems common in bicyclists are caused or aggravated by non-cycling activities such as running or weight training.

GENERAL ANATOMIC CLASSIFICATION OF OVERUSE INJURIES

Overuse injuries commonly affect four body structures: tendons, bursae, nerves, and bones.

Tendonitis

Tendons are fibrous cords of tissue that join muscles to bone. Tendonitis is inflammation or irritation of a tendon. See page 196 for further discussion.

Bursitis

Bursae are cystic structures between surfaces that move over each other, probably to lubricate movement. Sometimes the surface is a tendon, sometimes a bone. Bursitis is inflammation or irritation of a bursa. I cover bursitis in more detail on page 196.

Compression Neuropathy

A neuropathy is an abnormality of nerve function. Compression pressure on a nerve, or on the blood vessels that supply a nerve, is associated with several well-known neuropathies. Common cycling neuropathies include cyclist's palsy, a neuropathy of the ulnar nerve in the hand, and penile numbness, a common neuropathy related to abnormal function of the pudendal nerve.

Stress Fracture

A stress fracture is an overuse injury of bone. Beginning with microfractures, an untreated stress fracture may proceed to a completed, or through-and-through, fracture. Stress fractures are relatively uncommon in cycling.

Traumatic Injuries

Some traumatic, or sudden, injuries occur more frequently in cycling than in other sports. Other injuries are associated with cycling-specific treatments that allow athletes to return to riding sooner.

This book is not meant to be a comprehensive review of all traumatic injuries in cycling. Injuries that do occur in cyclists but occur with low frequency or are treated in the same way as in non-cyclists—such as splenic rupture or carpal bone fracture—will not be discussed.

GENERAL ANATOMIC CLASSIFICATION OF TRAUMATIC INJURIES

Traumatic injuries commonly affect ligaments (sprains and dislocations), tendons or muscles (strains), the skin (abrasions and lacerations), bones (fractures), and internal organs (contusions and lacerations).

Sprains

A sprain is a stretching injury to a ligament or group of ligaments (a ligament connects bone to bone, usually around a joint). First-degree sprains involve only excessive stretching, second-degree sprains are partial tears, and third-degree sprains are complete tears of ligaments. On examination, first-degree sprains have no abnormal laxity (looseness of the joint), and third-degree sprains have no end point (the ligament is not holding the joint together).

Stress X rays (X rays taken with weights pulling on the affected area or during manipulation of it) are often obtained to determine the severity of sprains, although many dispute their relevance, believing that clinical examination is at least as accurate. Although stress radiographs may confirm the diagnosis, such handling occasionally worsens the injury.

Third-degree sprains almost always require orthopedic consultation.

Strains

A strain is an injury to muscle or tendon. Often considered to be a stretching injury, a strain may also result from inappropriate internal tension—a slightly different concept. Some conceptualize an avulsion-type fracture to be a type of strain. First-degree strains involve only excessive stretching, second-degree strains are partial tears, and third-degree strains are complete tears. In young adults, these injuries usually occur at the muscle-tendon junction; in older individuals the tendon itself is usually the site of injury.

First-degree strains often occur over a series of muscle motions. The athlete may notice a pop or a snap with a single motion, signifying a second-degree strain. The dramatic pop or snap of a third-degree strain is often heard by others.

Internal Medical Problems

Several internal medical problems are caused by cycling. Other problems, though not caused by cycling, are worsened by it. Still others require modification or consideration in treatment because of cycling activities. Internal medical problems associated with cycling are discussed below.

Note on Anatomical Location and Terminology

Health professionals describe anatomical locations using a vocabulary foreign to many bicycle riders. In order to be understood by as wide an audience as possible, I've tried to use simple, consistent language when describing the anatomical location of medical problems. However, at times, precision is difficult without a specialized vocabulary.

Consider the knee. Does "inside" of the knee mean the side of the knee that the big toe is on, or does it mean where the joint surfaces rub against each other? I use the term *inside* to describe the medial surface, or side, and *internal* to describe the areas where the bones meet.

Road Rash

This most common of bicycling injuries can be treated in different ways. The right way reduces healing time and scarring, and allows you to return to your bike promptly.

Prevention

Learn bike handling skills to help prevent falling. Ride defensively, especially in traffic and around squirrelly riders. Always wear a helmet.

Treatment Objectives

The objective of treatment is to heal the tissues as rapidly and effectively as possible. The goals of therapy include preventing further damage to the skin and not allowing the depth of the rash to increase in severity.

What can go wrong? The rash can heal with scarring. The rash can take longer to heal than needed, because of infection, for example. Or the rash can heal well but be more painful than necessary during the healing process.

Grading Road Rash

The severity of road rash is similar to that of burns. Rash can be

- *First degree.* Only the surface is reddened. This problem does not require active treatment.
- *Second degree.* The surface layer of the skin is broken, but a deep layer remains that will allow the skin to replace itself and heal without significant scarring.
- *Third degree.* The skin is entirely removed, perhaps with exposure of underlying layers of fat and other supporting tissue structures. Such damage may require skin grafting and is beyond the scope of this book. Seek immediate medical attention.

Old-Style Treatment

There are two general methods of treatment for second-degree road rash. The first is the traditional "let nature take its course" approach, which is also called the open method. This involves cleaning the wound with soap and water, hydrogen peroxide, an iodide, or something similar, and then allowing the wound to dry out, form a scab, and "heal on its own."

This method has its drawbacks for all but the most superficial, small road rashes. Just because you clean it once doesn't mean it won't get infected. Bacteria thrive on damaged skin. Infection can deepen the depth of the rash, meaning that scarring and delayed healing are more likely. Scabs can crack and become painful. Scabbed areas don't receive oxygen well from the surrounding air, and so take much longer to heal.

Modern Thinking—Cover It

The alternative is the closed approach: frequent cleansings and the application of topical antibiotics and dressings that keep the road rash moist and closed to the air. The area is cleansed at least daily with wet compresses or bathing. Superficial debris is gently removed. An effort is made to remove soft-forming exudates (the beginnings of scabs) with gentle scrubbing. These exudates usually form between the third and fifth days after injury. Pink, healthy, new-forming skin is what you want to see. Second-degree road rash usually takes two to three weeks to heal.

Modern-Thinking Supplies

Silver sulfadiazine (Silvadene) or mupirocin (Bactroban) is applied. A Vaseline gauze (e.g., Adaptic) is placed over this. This is a non-stick mesh that allows removal of the dressing without sticking. Padding in the form of gauze squares may be applied. Then, a conforming gauze roll is wrapped around the area and taped in place. Finally, a tube stretch gauze (e.g., Tubigauze) is applied over this to keep everything in place and tidy. Alternatively, Tegaderm (3M) or Bioclusive (Johnson and Johnson) alone may be stretched over the antibiotic. The result is a dressing that allows maximum protection of the wound, minimum risk of infection, prevention of scabbing and its attendant cracking and pain, and fast healing.

Side Effects

Persons allergic to sulfa drugs should avoid sulfadiazine. Mupirocin is an alternative that are a little better at controlling skin infections, but it's more expensive. Neosporin or Polysporin is more likely to irritate the skin than sulfadiazine or mupirocin but are available over the counter.

Watch for Sunburn on Road Rash

As the skin nears complete healing you may be tempted to allow your technique to become lax. Exposure to sun may cause the skin to remain permanently darkened after healing. Be sure to keep your rash covered until it has completely healed. Use adequate (SPF >18) sunscreen.

Saddle Sores

Sores of the buttocks and groin area are a common occupational hazard for the bicycle rider. Many causes can be avoided. Specific treatment is available if saddle sores do develop.

What We're Talking About

The phrase *saddle sores* is used by different riders to refer to various separate problems involving the skin of the upper thigh and of the rear end. Pressure, friction, and infection are the three main causes of saddle sores.

FURUNCLES AND FOLLICULITIS

Blocked and/or infected glands and lumps are a common cycling problem. These painful bumps are classic saddle sores.

ISCHIAL TUBEROSITY PAIN

This is pain in the area of the pelvic bones that bear your weight on the bicycle seat. The ischial tuberosities are the "sitting bones." Occasionally, pain in this area progresses to either a local bursitis or ulceration.

CHAFING OF THE THIGH

Chafing of the inside of the upper leg is common in cyclists. It occurs because of friction caused by the repeated rubbing of the inside of the thigh during the up-and-down motion of the pedal stroke.

Many cyclists note that the insides of their shorts pill and wear with friction. When this happens to your inner thighs, redness and discomfort are the results. Dampness of the cycling shorts related to sweat production and the lack of breathability of the shorts' material may make the problem worse.

SKIN ULCERATION

Skin that is missing its topmost surface layers and denuded is ulcerated. This is sometimes an extreme result of rubbing or pressure.

RELATIVELY RARE PROBLEMS

- *Subcutaneous nodules.* These are a specific type of lump found in elite male cyclists near the scrotum, sometimes called "extra testicles."
- *Tailbone abscess.* A genetic predisposition to a blocked pilonidal sinus may be aggravated by cycling, and the sinus may become infected. Surgical treatment is often advised.

Saddle Sore Theory

There are two prevalent theories about the origin of classic saddle sores.

THE THREE CAUSES OF SADDLE SORES

- Infection
- Pressure
- Friction

The first has to do with infection and blocked glands. Bacteria get into glands and cause saddle sores. Therefore, treatment is directed at reducing the level of skin bacteria and preventing pore blockage.

The second theory has to do with pressure and friction. According to this theory, increased saddle pressure (which often arises through increased miles) prevents small blood vessels from bringing blood to the skin, and the skin gets fewer nutrients. This causes a breakdown in the skin's defenses, pore irritation, and blockage. Trapped bacteria may proliferate. A saddle sore develops.

Riders who always get saddle sores on the same cheek may find that the leg on that side is shorter. The buttock of a shorter leg gets more bumping and bruising.

Prevention

- Keep yourself dry. Modern synthetics wick away moisture and are softer on the skin than traditional leather chamois. Don't continue to wear wet sweat-drenched shorts after riding. Change into loose shorts that allow air to circulate. After bathing, allow your crotch to dry completely before putting on tight-fitting shorts or cycling shorts. Powder in your shorts can prevent chafing that may lead to irritation and infected blocked glands (although powder may be linked to some cervical problems in women).
- Keep yourself clean.
- Wear synthetic, padded cycling shorts.
- Always wear clean cycling shorts. Avoid wearing the same shorts two days in a row without laundering. Not only do soiled shorts have more bacteria, they don't breathe as well as freshly laundered ones.
- Avoid cycling shorts that have become pilled or that have seams in areas that either rub the inside thigh or upon which pressure is placed.
- Do not suddenly and drastically increase your weekly mileage.
- Use seats that provide enough padding to support, and spread the support over as wide an area as is compatible with your anatomy.
- Check your seat position.

- Avoid shaving above the shorts line to the groin. This often results in red spots caused by irritation and infection.

Self-Treatment

- Apply all the preventive measures described above.
- Modify your training. You don't have to stop cycling, but you may need to back off. This is not the time to increase mileage. A couple of years ago, when I had some bad saddle sores, I modified my routine. Tuesday was for hill sprints, Wednesday for long hill climbing, and Thursday for hill intervals—all done out of the saddle and off my sores!
- Soak in a comfortably hot bathtub three times a day for 15 minutes to allow boils to come to the surface and drain. Hot-water soaks increase blood circulation to the inflamed area, allowing more of the body's healing factors access to the area.
- For classic saddle sores or ischial tuberosity pain, pad your skin with padded tape or moleskin. You may want to reduce the tackiness of moleskin by first applying it to something other than your skin. Leave some tack so that it will still stick, but not so much that it pulls your skin and hair off when you remove it later.
- Another possibility is to take a couple of Band-Aids or a layer of moleskin and cut out a small hole for the sore, effectively padding around the sore and taking pressure off the sore itself.
- The extra padding of a second pair of shorts worn over the first may help.
- A padded seat cover may help.
- A different seat may help.
- Suspension may help. Rear-end suspension or beamed seat tubes reduce saddle pressure.
- A modification of seat position—nose up or down, forward or back, up or down—may help.
- Friction-related problems may be helped by an emollient, such as Vaseline.
- Topical cortisone, antifungal, and antibacterial creams may help.
- Some riders swear by a veterinary product called Bag Balm.
- Shimming the shoe of the shorter leg may help if saddle sores are related to leg length discrepancy.

Medical and Surgical Treatment

- If the area around the sore is infected, it may require surgical drainage or antibiotics.
- Uninfected sores that remain as painful, swollen, hard lumps can occasionally be treated with a cortisone injection.
- Occasionally surgery may be required to remove chronic cysts.

Crotchitis

Crotchitis is irritation or inflammation of the crotch. Redness, itching, and pain are problems in this area. Crotchitis is common in women—specifically, irritation of the skin around the vagina, the clitoris, and the urethra. Crotchitis is distinctive from saddle sores, discussed in the previous section.

Prevention

The best treatment is prevention. Some general measures will help almost all cases of crotchitis. Some treatments may improve some cases of crotchitis but may actually make other cases worse! It is therefore important to determine the cause of your crotchitis.

Causes of Crotchitis

Many cases of crotchitis are related to a combination of factors:

- Warmth
- Moisture
- Hygienic practices and irritants
- Friction
- Bicycle position and saddle
- Medical problems, including dermatitis
- Allergy
- Vaginal infections

Warmth and Moisture

Warmth and moisture aggravate most cases of crotchitis. Avoid traveling to races or rides in your car already wearing your bike shorts. Change into bike shorts when you arrive. Use bike shorts with a breathable, moisture-wicking crotch. Change out of moist or wet bicycling shorts as soon as possible after riding. Wear loose-fitting shorts or a skirt. Wear breathable fabrics and cotton underwear. Avoid tight-fitting non-breathing underwear, or wear no underwear. Pantyhose is an enemy of the crotch.

Allow ventilation to cool and dry the area. Avoid sitting on non-breathing surfaces such as plastic and leather. Use a car seat cover with air holes if your car has vinyl or leather seats.

YEAST OVERGROWTH—JOCK ITCH, CROTCH ROT

Moisture and warmth cause yeast overgrowth, commonly called jock itch or crotch rot. Over-the-counter antifungal creams and powders may help reduce yeast overgrowth. Occasionally irritated skin can also be helped by over-the-counter cortisone cream, although cortisone sometimes worsens yeast overgrowth.

Hygiene and Irritants

Stool is a powerful irritant. Clean yourself properly. Overzealous hygiene can be just as much of a problem as lack of hygiene. When you are irritated, wiping and rubbing can cause chafing and further irritation. Since this area always has some bacteria, and since irritated skin is prone to worsen and get infected, overzealous wiping must be avoided. Avoid wiping affected areas with rough toilet tissue. Wipe from front to back. Women, don't carry bacteria toward your vagina and urethra. Not only will this worsen crotchitis, but urinary tract infections and vaginal infections may result as well.

Avoid local irritants such as harsh soaps.

If crotchitis extends to areas you need to wipe to keep clean, consider using facial tissue, gentle medicated over-the-counter products such as Tucks, moistened toilet paper, or plain water. Clean, and then pat—not wipe—dry.

Friction

Friction can be minimized by using an emollient skin preparation, such as Vaseline, or an anti-yeast cream. A seat pad or cover fitted over your saddle may allow slight movement and function in the same way as a sock in a shoe. Wearing two pairs of lightweight bicycling shorts or a lightweight bicycling liner may help to reduce friction-caused crotchitis. However, if crotchitis is related to warmth and moisture, doubling up on your shorts may make things worse.

Bicycle Position

Most bicycles are sized for men, making the top tube stem length too long for most women even if the frame fits otherwise. This puts extra pressure on the crotch. Make sure your bicycle position is not too stretched out.

Saddle

Saddle position and saddle type may be factors relating to crotchitis. Consider the seat angle. A slight nose-down position may help, especially for time trial events or crits when you are in an aerodynamic position and putting a lot of pressure on the crotch. Some women prefer a nose-up position so that the saddle presses more on the pubic bone and less on the soft tissues around the vagina.

Move around frequently, and get off that saddle when you can. Stand up on your pedals to relieve crotch friction and pressure. When climbing hills, stand up periodically. When descending, put weight on your pedals and get off your crotch. This allows moving air to cool and dry your crotch while you relieve pressure. If you are riding tandem, be sure to take frequent crotch breaks by getting out of the saddle at stop signs and stop lights and by standing out of the saddle with your partner at least every 15 minutes.

Terry saddles have padding and are less stiff. Many women report that although these saddles feel no different from other saddles while they are riding, at the end of a ride their crotches don't hurt as much. Severe cases of crotchitis may require drastic measures—cutting or paring your seat may be necessary to keep riding.

Allergies

Many riders use a wide variety of products on their skin that may cause allergies. For example, to help with saddle sores near the crotch, riders may use tapes or pads to which they may have a tape allergy. This worsens saddle sores into saddle sores plus crotchitis! Some riders use perfumed or chemically treated products such as sprays, sanitary napkins, or lubricating oils to which they may be allergic. These can then cause or worsen crotchitis.

Vaginal Infections

The extra moisture related to a vaginal infection may worsen crotchitis. Treating the underlying vaginal discharge may help improve crotchitis. Infected or otherwise blocked sweat or other glands may develop into crotchitis if friction worsens these conditions.

Other Infections

Occasionally other infections, such as herpes, cause crotch irritation. In turn, crotch irritation can also promote or exacerbate herpes outbreaks in people who harbor the virus.

Medical Problems

Riders with skin conditions such as psoriasis or eczema may have flare-ups in this area related to friction and other general factors listed above. Prescription-strength cortisone creams are often the best help for these problems. Occasionally other medical problems such as lactose intolerance or pinworms are the cause.

Neck and Back Pain

Neck Pain

WHAT WE'RE TALKING ABOUT

Pain in the back of the neck that may or may not travel upward and cause headache. See a doctor whenever neck pain is associated with loss of sensation, loss of power, or pain in your arms. Pain in the front of the neck or in the jaw associated with exercise can originate from the heart. See a doctor if you experience this kind of pain.

CAUSES

Neck pain can be a result of strain or overuse. The pain may travel to the back of the head and become more generalized. If nerves are involved, it may travel to the arms. It is usually due to one of these causes:

- Muscle strain and/or spasm.
- Arthritis—usually wear-and-tear/degenerative arthritis, or osteoarthritis. Strain on the vertebral joints from misalignment, often secondary to disc degeneration, also causes pain.
- A bulge or herniation of an intervertebral disc. This may cause pain that travels to the arms. If you have arm symptoms associated with neck pain, see a doctor.

In younger cyclists, neck pain is usually due to muscle strain. In older cyclists, a combination of muscle strain and degenerative changes is often responsible. Degenerative—wear-and-tear—changes are aging-related, not cycling-related.

Cycling-related neck strain is often associated with long rides.

Position on the bike can be a factor. Cyclists lacking flexibility may find the aerodynamic bent-over racing position uncomfortable. Anything that forces the rider to increase stretch in the neck may cause neck pain. For example, women tend to ride bikes with top tubes that are too long for them, since most bikes are designed for men. Women have relatively longer legs and relatively shorter reaches.

Jarring from rough mountain bike riding can be a factor, although road rides are worse for riders who forget to look around.

Neck pain may additionally be non–cycling-related, arising from

- Muscle tension due to stress, anxiety, depression, or fatigue
- Poor posture

TREATMENT

On the Bicycle

If your problem is due to long rides:

- Allow for a gradual increase in endurance riding. Increase the length of endurance rides no more than 10% per week.
- Consciously relax your upper body—back, elbows, and neck—every few minutes. Changing hand positions will change neck position and in turn reduce strain.
- Stretch your neck on the bike. Look around—don't focus only on the pavement directly in front of you.
- A helmet is a must for safety—but make sure yours is lightweight.

If your problem comes from craning your neck on the bike:

- Ride with a more upright posture.
- Ride on the hoods or tops of the handlebars. Avoid the drops. Use a more upright bar.
- Reduce the distance you need to stretch. Raise or shorten the stem. Use narrower handlebars. Get a bike with a shorter top tube.

If your problem is due to jarring:

- Get a gel saddle.
- Use padded gloves or padded handlebars or grips.
- Use a suspension system.

- Use wider tires.
- Ride a mountain bike on road rides.
- Use lower tire pressure.
- Consider a recumbent bike.

Off the Bicycle

R.I.C.E. Discussed on page 167.

Strengthening. Strengthening the neck muscles may help. Do not work on these muscle groups while you are still injured. Isometric neck exercises are helpful: use your hand to resist the motion of your head up-and-down and side-to-side. Shoulder shrugs are helpful.

Stretching. Helps some people. Voluntary range of motion exercises may help increase the flexibility of your neck. Avoid active range of motion exercises with machines, weights, or forcing your neck into positions—they may result in injury.

NSAIDs. Anti-inflammatory pain medicines are useful and are discussed on page 161.

Surgery. Usually the last-resort treatment. A surgical emergency may exist if the nerves being pinched in the neck interfere with muscle sensation or power elsewhere in the body.

Chiropractic Manipulation. Symptomatically helps some people with pain, although many traditional physicians dispute its effectiveness.

Scapula Syndrome

WHAT WE'RE TALKING ABOUT

Pain in the upper back, around the shoulder blade. It may or may not be associated with neck, shoulder, or arm symptoms. It may or may not be related to cycling. It overlaps with neck ache, discussed above.

CYCLING-RELATED CAUSES OF SCAPULA SYNDROME

- Extended saddle time. The longer you are in the saddle, the more time other factors act to increase tension in this area.
- Rough terrain and jarring.

- Too much pressure. Weight distribution too far forward puts more pressure on the upper back and neck.
- Excessive use of upper back and neck muscles during sprinting, climbing, or other efforts.

MEDICAL CAUSES

The pain may be due to a muscular problem or a pinched nerve. Cycling related problems are due to overuse or strain. Non–cycling-related causes include pulls or strains, muscular tension related to stress or depression, arthritis, and posture. If scapula pain is associated with pain that travels down the arm, is more than mild, or persists for more than two weeks, medical attention is advised.

TREATMENT

On the Bicycle

- Reduce mileage:
  Readapt slowly.
- Prevent jarring:
  Use padded gloves.
  Use padded handlebar tape or grips.
  Try suspension.
- Reduce pressure:
  Sit more upright.
  Vary your position.
  Raise the stem height.
  Check that your seat is not too far forward.
  Use a shorter stem.
  Avoid tilting the saddle down.
  Use a shorter top tube.
- Avoid strain:
  Reduce hard efforts involving the upper back muscles.

Off the Bicycle

While you are symptomatic, avoid offending activities, including upper body work and excessive time looking at video screens.

Medical Treatment

R.I.C.E. Local applications of ice may be helpful. If the problem relates to a pinched nerve in the neck, a neck collar may be helpful.

Strengthening. Strengthening of the neck, arms, and upper back may be helpful.

Stretching. Improving neck and back flexibility may be helpful.

Massage. It may be helpful.

NSAIDs. Useful, and discussed on page 161.

Cortisone. Rarely used in this location, although injections of anesthetics, or "numbing medicines," can be tried.

Surgery. The treatment of last resort, used only if the cause is related to a pinched nerve.

Low Back Pain

WHAT WE'RE TALKING ABOUT

Low back ache that makes riding uncomfortable. Pain that forces you to slow down or get off the bike. See a doctor whenever back pain is associated with loss of sensation or power in your legs.

CAUSES

Back Strain

Acute low back pain can follow strain or overuse. The pain may travel to the buttock or thigh, but if nerves are not involved, it does not travel below the knee. It is usually due to

- Muscle strain and/or spasm.
- Arthritis—usually wear-and-tear/degenerative arthritis, or osteoarthritis. Strain on the vertebral joints from misalignment, often secondary to disc degeneration, also causes pain.
- A bulge or herniation of an intervertebral disc. This is discussed more under "Nerve Compression," below.

In younger cyclists, back pain is usually due to muscle strain. In older cyclists, a combination of muscle strain and degenerative changes is usually responsible. Cycling-related back strain is often related to long rides, big gears, or hill work. Big-gear riding and hill climbing—especially on long grades—results in back pain because riders tighten their back muscles to get more power.

Position on the bike can be important. Cyclists lacking flexibility may find the aerodynamic bent-over racing position uncomfortable. Anything that forces the rider to increase stretch may cause back pain.

Jarring from rough riding can be a factor.

Chronic low back pain may additionally be due to non–cycling-related factors, such as

- Leg-length difference
- Swayback
- Deconditioning and poor posture
- Muscle tension due to stress, anxiety, depression, or fatigue

Nerve Compression—"Pinched Nerve"

The spinal cord travels down inside the spine, or vertebral column. The vertebrae are cushioned, one from the other, by discs composed of fiber-like and jelly-like material. The spinal nerves exit between the bones of the spine, or vertebrae. Sometimes the nerves are pinched by a disc, which has been squeezed out of position between two vertebrae, or by the bones themselves.

The spinal nerves of the lower back form the sciatic nerve, which travels down the buttocks area and the back of the thigh. The various component spinal nerves then travel to various parts of the leg.

Nerves have pain sensors; other sensory fibers; and motor, or muscle-moving, fibers. The progression of severity of pinched nerves is usually pain, sensory change, and muscle weakness, in that order. Sensory changes include a pins-and-needle sensation, tingling, and areas of numbness.

When a nerve is being pinched, symptoms may occur along the area supplied by the nerve. Pain that radiates from the buttocks down the back of the thighs is commonly called sciatica. Pinched nerves in the back are the most frequent, but not the only, cause of sciatica. Occasionally the nerve is pinched in a buttock muscle, the piriformis, rather than in the spine.

Obtain consultation with a physician whenever you experience sensory change or muscle weakness.

TREATMENT

On the Bicycle

If your problem is due to excessive exercise load:

- Allow for a gradual increase in endurance riding. Increase the length of endurance rides no more than 10% per week.
- If big gears are in your training program, allow yourself to adapt to them slowly.

If your problem is due to hills:

- Reduce hill mileage and then adapt to increased mileage slowly.
- Shift your position every so often from seated to standing. Consciously relax your back every few minutes when climbing.
- Take a rest break at the side of the road on long climbs. Enjoy the view!

If your problem is a too stretched-out position on the bike:

- Reduce stretch by assuming a more upright posture. Ride on the hoods or tops of the handlebars.
- Reduce the distance you need to stretch. Raise or shorten the stem. Use narrower handlebars. Get a bike with a shorter top tube.

If buttock pain or sciatica is related to nerve pressure in the piriformis muscle:

- Get a gel-filled or a more compliant saddle.

If your problem is due to jarring:

- Get a gel saddle.
- Use wider tires.
- Use a rear suspension system.
- Use lower tire pressure.
- Ride a mountain bike on road rides.
- Consider a recumbent bike.

Off the Bicycle

R.I.C.E. Discussed more fully on page 167. Studies show that even the worst strains require, at most, a few days of bed rest. Mild strains may disappear as soon as you are off the bike. Ice or heat may help.

Strengthening. Strengthening the back and abdominal muscles may help. Do not work on these muscles while you are still injured. Climbing or gradually increasing mileage will often adapt the body sufficiently. Bent knee sit-ups, crunches, back extensions, pelvic tilt exercises, and rowing strengthen the back and abdominals.

Stretching. Helps some people. Back flexion exercises are most helpful. In individuals who have lost the normal curve, giving a flat back, extension exercises are more useful. Hamstring stretching relieves some of the need for the back to bend, and can help.

NSAIDs. Anti-inflammatory pain medicines are useful and are discussed on page 161.

Orthotics. A heel lift or cleat shim may help if a leg length difference exists.

Surgery. Usually the last-resort treatment. A surgical emergency exists if the nerves being pinched interfere with bowel or bladder function, or if rapidly progressive leg weakness occurs.

Weight Loss: Lessens back pain in many who are overweight.

Chiropractic Manipulation: Symptomatically helps many with back pain, although many traditional physicians dispute its effectiveness.

Posture Hints for Low Back Pain

- Sit or stand using a footrest to bend the knee and hip of one leg.
- Lie either curled up on your side, or on your back with pillows under your knees. Do not lie on your belly. When rising from a lying position, roll to your side and push yourself up with your arm.
- Bend from the hips and knees; avoid bending from the waist.
- Carry or lift only what you can handle with ease.
- Turn and face the object you wish to lift.
- Hold heavy objects close to your body.
- Avoid lifting heavy objects higher than your waist.
- Avoid carrying unbalanced loads.
- Avoid sudden movements.
- Change positions frequently.
- Work with tools close to the body. Avoid long reaches when raking, hoeing, mopping, or vacuuming.
- Sit down to dress. Bend your leg when putting on shoes and socks; do not bend from the waist.
- Wear low heels.

Tendonitis and Bursitis

What Is Tendonitis?

Tendons are fibrous cords of tissue that join muscles to bone. Tendonitis is inflammation or irritation of a tendon.

Tendons allow the muscles to move bones relative to each other at the joints. Irritation to a tendon can have different causes. A fall may bruise a tendon; overuse may strain a tendon; sudden forces or extra hard efforts may do the same. Pain comes from nerve irritation within the tendon and is a warning sign that something is wrong—the tendon itself may be stretched and swollen, or small parts of it may actually be torn.

What Is Bursitis?

Bursae are cystic structures that form between surfaces that move over each other, probably to lubricate movement. Sometimes the surface is a tendon, sometimes a bone. Bursitis is inflammation or irritation of a bursa.

When one of the surfaces is a tendon, it is often impossible to distinguish between tendonitis and bursitis. The difference between tendonitis and bursitis in such a situation may be of little relevance, since the treatment of both conditions is often the same.

Normal Healing

Most injuries of this type heal themselves within a few days. Avoiding further injury to this area by resting is the traditional treatment. Conservative doctors may advise complete cessation of the activity that produced the injury.

Several things are going on. One is that the tendon is injured and needs to repair itself. The other is that the body's mechanism of warning that this repair process must be heeded can be an overcompensation of inflammation. Slight tearing of microscopic parts of the tendon may not be significant; however, the body's response—excessive local irritation—may be your biggest problem.

Modify Your Riding

I agree that modified rest is important. However, it may be safe to continue cycling, as long as you avoid excessive strain on the tendon involved. Read "Ride or Rest?" on page 170.

Anti-Inflammatory Medicine

If the problem is related to excessive inflammation, you can reduce it with NSAIDs (anti-inflammatory medicines). Anti-inflammatory medicines form the cornerstone of medical treatment of tendonitis. Read more about anti-inflammatories on page 161.

Other Treatments

There are other forms of therapy apart from rest and aspirin. You may have a biomechanical problem that requires fundamental correction. For example, you may have a tendonitis around your knee because your shoe cleat is improperly placed.

Sometimes physical therapy, though expensive, may be helpful. For some cases of tendonitis, a cortisone shot can work wonders.

Seek Help

It is usually safe to try modified rest and an anti-inflammatory on your own for a couple of weeks before consulting a doctor. With persistent problems, medical advice may prove helpful.

Upper Extremity

Broken Collarbone

COMMON BREAK

The collarbone is the most common bone to break when a cyclist falls. It is usually the result of falling on an outstretched hand, which causes indirect violence to the shoulder girdle. You can easily feel your clavicle (collarbone) running from the sternum (breastplate bone) to the acromion, a projection forward from the scapula (shoulder blade).

HEALING

Most bones heal or "knit" in about six weeks. The collarbone is no exception. As the collarbone heals it forms callus, or "bone glue," where it was broken.

This callus results in a thickened area. In many, the collarbone is actually stronger after it heals than it was before it was broken.

About 80% of the time, the collarbone breaks about where the middle third meets the outer third. This type of collarbone fracture, when the bones are in good alignment, has an excellent prognosis. About 15% of the time, the break occurs very close to the shoulder at the acromioclavicular (A-C) joint, in which case healing may be more difficult. Rarely does a break occur near the sternum, or breastplate.

Most collarbone injuries will heal well without much medical or surgical intervention. A figure-of-eight bandage, which pulls the shoulders back, is sometimes prescribed for a couple of weeks. This may help keep the ends of the break in better alignment and reduce discomfort. Although most physicians prescribe a figure-of-eight bandage routinely, surprisingly few believe that it actually does much good. Additionally, the arm is often placed in a sling. Most patients discard the sling and bandage after a week or two.

Occasionally the bones do not "knit," or form good callus, but heal loosely with only a fibrous connection. Surgery may be required in the unusual case when a collarbone injury does not heal on its own. Occasionally the break compresses a nerve, and surgery is required for decompression. Surgery may be advisable from the outset in some breaks close to the A-C joint associated with significant tearing of ligaments.

Pain relief is discussed on page 163.

RETURN TO RIDING

For aligned collarbone breaks in a very motivated athlete, when normal healing is expected, training can resume almost immediately, usually in forty-eight hours. Since jarring from the road is uncomfortable, training is performed on a stationary trainer. A specific workout plan is invaluable—otherwise, most riders piddle away their time on the trainer without productive work. Raising the front of the trainer slightly and/or raising the nose of the saddle slightly will allow the rider to ride in a more upright position with less weight on the shoulder and less pain.

Active shoulder exercises may be begun when pain lessens, usually about one week after injury. Most riders with fractured collarbones can ride the road in about two weeks, especially with a hybrid or mountain bike with fat tires that absorb road shock. Serious road riding and racing can resume, if all goes well, in four to six weeks. Mountain bike racing may be delayed another month.

The above are guidelines for motivated racers with "good" breaks. One rider from our club won a National Championship a week after his collarbone was fractured. Some riders take several months to get back into the swing of things.

Shoulder Separation—A-C Sprain

WHAT WE'RE TALKING ABOUT

Shoulder separation, and acromioclavicular (A-C) sprain, are terms for a stretching or tearing of the shoulder ligaments. The collarbone meets the shoulder blade at the acromioclavicular joint. This is a forward-pointing prominence of the outside (lateral aspect) of the shoulder blade.

The clavicle is held to the shoulder blade at the A-C joint by a fibrous envelope, or capsule. There are also two coracoclavicular ligaments—fibrous attachments between the clavicle and the coracoid part of the shoulder blade.

In cycling, injuries to this area by direct trauma are common. Falls tend to force the acromion downward, stretching or tearing it (and the rest of the shoulder blade) away from the collarbone.

SEVERITY OF INJURY

Shoulder separations are graded by severity and by their appearance on X ray. X rays are sometimes taken with weights on the affected arm to help show any weakness of the structures.

GRADING SHOULDER SEPARATION SEVERITY

- *First-degree separation.* The capsule of the A-C joint is stretched but not completely torn. There is local pain at the A-C joint, which worsens with abduction (raising outward) of the arm. X rays do not show any movement at the A-C joint.

Figure 4-1

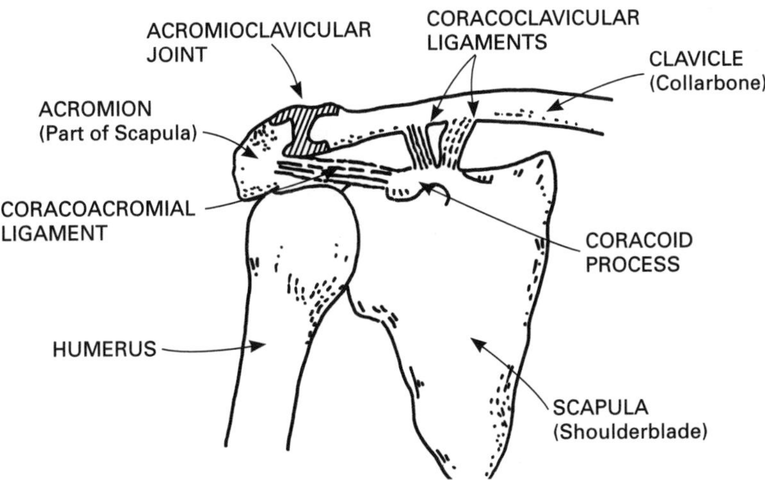

The shoulder joint area, front view. A shoulder separation is a stretching or tearing of the shoulder ligaments.

- *Second-degree separation.* Capsule disruption is such that X ray shows some movement of the acromion downward relative to the clavicle. This displacement is less than the width of the clavicle.
- *Third-degree separation.* The separation is as much as, or more than, the width of the clavicle. The coracoclavicular ligaments have been torn. An operation may be necessary.

TREATMENT

First- and second-degree separations are treated with a sling. Range of motion exercises may begin when pain allows, usually within a week of the injury. Stationary trainer workouts may begin almost immediately. Road riding and racing can commence as discomfort allows. Third-degree separations may take as long as six weeks to heal.

Pain relief is discussed below.

Shoulder Dislocation

The head of the humerus occasionally pops out of its socket. Dislocations may be associated with chipped bones or other fractures, ligament damage, nerve involvement, or damage to blood vessels. Dislocations of the shoulder are usually put back into place in the emergency room. A sling is often prescribed for discomfort. Pain in uncomplicated dislocations subsides quickly.

Although training on a stationary trainer may resume almost immediately, many physicians believe that keeping the arm in a sling for three weeks, together with physical therapy, helps prevent recurrent dislocations.

Shoulder Injury Pain Relief

Pain after shoulder injuries is normally worst during the first forty-eight hours. Most pain subsides after two or three weeks. Pain at night and difficulty finding a comfortable sleeping position is an expected problem.

There is controversy about the best medicine to use for pain. Non-steroidal anti-inflammatory drugs (NSAIDs) are the most commonly prescribed class of medicines. They have pain-relieving properties as well as anti-inflammatory ones. Some may be irritating to the gastrointestinal tract. Over-the-counter medications that fall into this class include plain aspirin, ibuprofen (Advil, Motrin) and naproxen (Aleve). Read more about anti-inflammatories on page 161.

Although anti-inflammatories are the most commonly used medicines for pain relief, some medical evidence suggests that they might delay bone healing. Some authorities avoid anti-inflammatories for this reason.

For the first few days, stronger relief with narcotics may be helpful. Tylenol with codeine is frequently prescribed. This combination affords better pain relief than most NSAIDs, but it is not anti-inflammatory, and it is also constipating and sedating. Switch away from narcotics as soon as possible.

Shoulder Injury Exercises

Although some guidelines are given in the discussion of specific injuries above, consult with your physician before beginning shoulder injury exercises.

PENDULUM EXERCISES

Do these with about 5 pounds of weight in your hand. Exercises can be done while you are standing and leaning over, but ideally do them on a bench, facing downwards, supporting yourself with your good arm.

- Move your arm forward and backward; allow the weight in your hand to help you swing as far as you can.
- Do the same thing side-to-side.
- Make circles in one direction, wider and wider; then go in the other direction.

WALL CLIMBING

- Face the wall with your outstretched hand and with your fingertips just touching the wall. Walk your fingertips up the wall. You will gradually and slowly walk toward the wall as your fingertips travel higher. Repeat ten times.
- Do the same thing standing sideways to the wall. Starting with your fingertips near your side, move slightly away from the wall to allow your fingers to creep up to the horizontal. As they rise above the horizontal, you will need to approach the wall again.

Weak Arms

Many cyclists complain that their arms get weak, especially during long descents or during hard, time-trialing–like efforts when their arms are in the drops.

The reason is usually weak triceps. The solution is a strengthening program to increase triceps strength. Triceps presses or dips are suitable exercises.

Elbow Pain

WHAT WE'RE TALKING ABOUT

Pain at either the inside or the outside of the elbow, unrelated to sudden injury. Injury, fracture, and swelling of the elbow are not discussed here. Consult a physician if these problems are present.

Figure 4-2

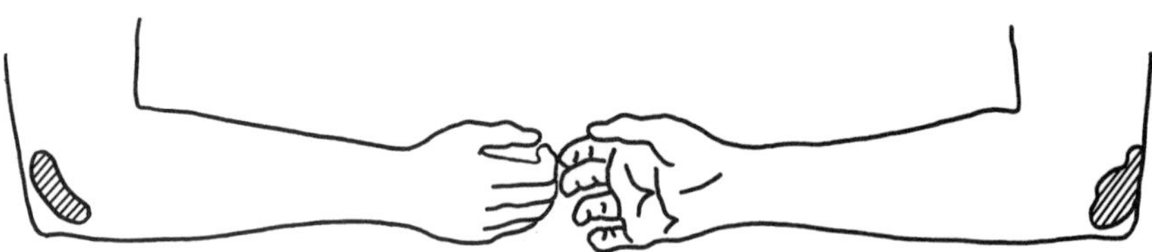

Lateral Epicondylitis
"Tennis Elbow"

Medial Epicondylitis

CAUSES

Repetitive twisting usually causes the problem. The twisting irritates the muscles that travel to and attach near the elbow. The irritation is often accompanied by microtears of the tendons. Pain at the outside of the elbow is lateral epicondylitis, or "tennis elbow." Pain at the inside is medial epicondylitis, "reverse tennis elbow." Tennis *is* a frequent cause, but any repetitive twisting motion—whether it be polishing doorknobs, sorting items into slots, painting, or shaking hands—can cause the problem. Cycling-related elbow pain is most frequent in mountain bikers who repetitively twist gear and brake levers. It may also occur in cyclists who ride tensed-up with rigid outstretched arms.

TREATMENT

On the Bicycle

Be aware of twisting motions. Use a setup that reduces your need to twist or that places the shifters and brakes in a more ergonomic position.

Off the Bicycle

Avoid other offending activities.

Medical Treatment

R.I.C.E. A so-called tennis-elbow band or support may be helpful. These come in a variety of forms, but the key is a non-elastic strapping about one-inch wide placed about one inch below your elbow. This helps stabilize the muscles that attach to your elbow. Locally applied ice may be helpful.

Massage. May be helpful. A special technique used in this area is friction massage.

Stretching. Specific stretches discussed and shown on page 150 may be useful.

NSAIDs. Useful, and discussed on page 161.

Cortisone. May be helpful.

Surgery. This is the treatment of last resort.

Cyclist's Palsy—Ulnar Neuropathy

WHAT WE'RE TALKING ABOUT

Pain, tingling, numbness, and weakness in the hand along the course of the ulnar nerve. The symptoms usually manifest themselves in the pinky and ring fingers and are worse during riding or for several hours after. Although this problem usually improves after riding stops, it can lead to permanent nerve injury if ignored.

Figure 4-3

Ulnar nerve pathway in the hand

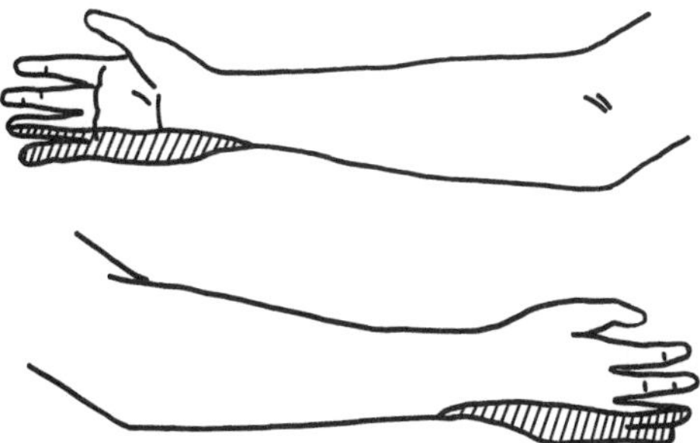

CAUSES

The ulnar nerve in the heel of the hand (the fleshy part of the hand below the pinky) is compressed.

Cycling-related causes include

- Extended saddle time. The longer you are in the saddle, the more time other factors act to press on the hand.
- Rough terrain; jarring of the hands while gripping the handlebars.
- Improper hand position. Too much time on the tops with the heel of the hand pressed against the bar.
- Too much pressure. Weight distribution too far forward puts more pressure on the hands, wrists, and arms.

The affected hand is usually the one that stays on the handlebar—the one that doesn't reach for the water bottle.

TREATMENT

On the Bicycle

Keep pressure off the heel of the affected hand when riding.

- Reduce mileage:
  Readapt slowly.
- Prevent jarring:
  Use padded or gel gloves.
  Use wider tires.
  Use padded, even double, handlebar tape, or padded grips.
  Use lower tire pressure.
  Try suspension.
- Improve hand position:
  Reposition your hands frequently.
  Relax your hands, wrists, and upper body.
- Reduce pressure:
  Avoid placing pressure on the heel of your hand.
  Vary your position.
  Raise the stem height.
  Check that your seat is not too far forward.
  Use a shorter stem.
  Avoid tilting the saddle down.
  Use a shorter top tube.

Medical Treatment

NSAIDs. May be helpful, but the best approach is to get pressure off the heel of your hand when riding. Read more about anti-inflammatories on page 161.

Carpal Tunnel Syndrome

WHAT WE'RE TALKING ABOUT

Pain, tingling, numbness, and weakness in the hand along the course of the median nerve. Symptoms may be present in the thumb, index, middle, and ring fingers and may also travel above the wrist to the elbow and shoulder. Symptoms are often worse at night.

Figure 4-4

Median nerve pathway in the hand

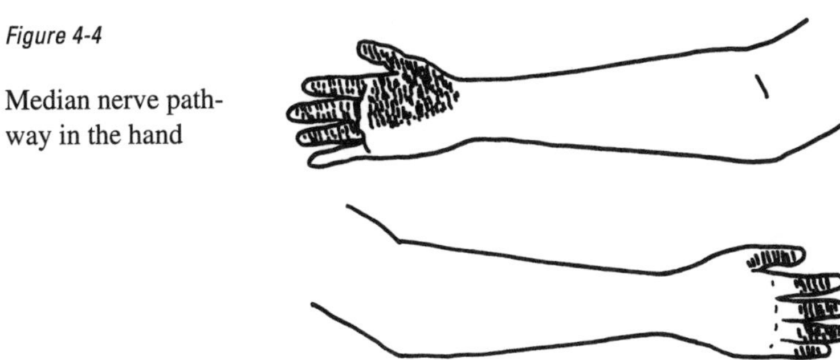

CAUSES

The median nerve is compressed in the wrist. Compression is usually due to inflammation. This problem is common in those who repeatedly bend their wrists on the job. Grocery checkers and keyboard operators, for example, have a high incidence of this problem. It can also be associated with medical conditions such as diabetes and pregnancy.

CYCLING-RELATED CAUSES OF CARPAL TUNNEL SYNDROME

- Extended saddle time. The longer you are in the saddle, the more time other factors act to increase inflammation in the wrist. The swelling then presses on the nerve.
- Rough terrain. Jarring of the wrists, especially while mountain biking, increases inflammation.
- Improper wrist position. Unnatural bending of the wrist while holding the handlebar predisposes to this problem.
- Too much pressure. Weight distribution too far forward puts more pressure on the hands, wrists, and arms.

TREATMENT

On the Bicycle

- Reduce mileage:
  Readapt slowly.
- Prevent jarring:
  Use padded gloves.
  Use wider tires.
  Use padded handlebar tape, or padded grips.
  Use lower tire pressure.
  Try suspension.
- Improve wrist position:
  Reposition your hands frequently.
  Relax your wrists and upper body.
  Make sure your handlebars are the correct width.
- Reduce pressure:
  Avoid placing undue pressure on the problem wrist. The affected hand is usually the one that stays on the handlebar—the one that doesn't reach for the water bottle.
  Vary your position.
  Raise the stem height.
  Check that your seat is not too far forward.
  Use a shorter stem.
  Avoid tilting the saddle down.
  Use a shorter top tube.

Off the Bicycle

Reduce repetitive motion at work or elsewhere.

Medical Treatment

R.I.C.E. A wrist rest, in the form of wrist braces or splints, is very helpful. Braces are worn at night or around the clock.

Strengthening. Strengthening the wrists, arms, and shoulders can help provide muscular support when you are riding, reducing pressure on the wrist.

NSAIDs. Helpful. See anti-inflammatories on page 161.

Cortisone. Can be used in this location.

Surgery. To increase the space around the nerve. A common operation when the above methods fail.

Finger Bumps

WHAT WE'RE TALKING ABOUT

Inflammation—swelling, discomfort, pain, or redness—at the side of the knuckles, which commonly results from pressure or friction between the bone and the handlebar. Sometimes the problem is caused by a non–cycling-related arthritis.

TREATMENT

If cycling-related, reduce the pressure or friction:

- Change hand positions to avoid pressure or friction.
- Make sure that bicycle fit gives good weight distribution without undue hand pressure.
- Use padded gloves or handlebar tape.

Pelvic Fracture

The Pelvic Ring

The pelvis forms a solid ring composed of three bones: the two hip bones in the front and sides, and the sacrum in the back. A hip bone has three regions—the ilium (side and back part), the ischium (with the hip socket and "sit" bone), and the pubis (the front part). The pubis itself has a top and bottom attachment to the other parts of the hip bone—the superior (above) and inferior (below) pubic rami.

Since the pelvis forms a solid ring, or circle, one break in the circle doesn't result in movement of the ring. It takes two breaks, usually on opposite sides of the pelvis, for the bones to separate. Figure 4-5 demonstrates isolated and displaced fractures.

Common Pelvic Breaks

Fractures of the superior (above) and inferior (below) pubic rami are the most common pelvic fractures. Fractures of the superior and inferior pubic rami, although really two fractures, count as "only one," since they basically disrupt only one part of the pubic ring.

Figure 4-5

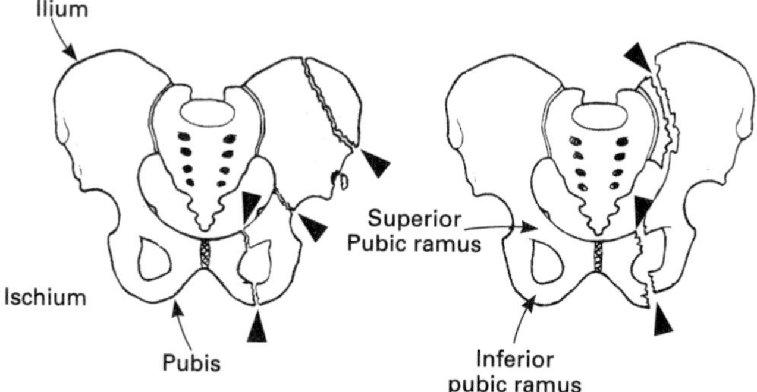

Pelvic injuries.
Isolated pelvic fractures, as in any one of the injuries on the left, leave the pelvic ring intact. They require only simple treatment. When multiple breaks are present at once, as on the right, the pelvic ring is unstable. Treatment is complex.

Treatment

No special treatment is usually needed for these common, single-fracture injuries, except to relieve pain. Rest for two or three weeks is usually enough. The treatment of multiple breaks is complex and individualized.

Complications

The bladder or urethra (urine tube from the bladder through the penis or vulva) may be damaged.

Bruising is expected. Blood in the tissues often follows the "path of least resistance"—i.e., gravity. Since there's a lot of room in the genital area for blood to collect, expect bruising (and later yellow and green discoloration) to develop in these areas even if actual injury did not occur here.

Return to Cycling

Leg exercises and cycling as tolerated on a stationary trainer can be started as soon as one feels comfortable enough to proceed.

Don't expect to compete for at least one month.

Lower Extremity

Leg-Length Discrepancy

WHAT WE'RE TALKING ABOUT

Many riders have legs of different lengths. This usually doesn't cause problems, especially if the difference is slight. But leg-length discrepancy *can* be a cause of leg or back discomfort. Traditionally, differences less than ¼ inch (or 6 millimeters) are not considered significant. Some have claimed that differences of as little as ⅛ inch (or 3 millimeters) are significant.

Although some theorize that correcting leg-length discrepancy results in a more effective stroke, I know of no studies that have ever shown that it improves power or aerobic economy. Shims, other devices, and cleat positioning can correct for leg-length discrepancy and can help these discomforts.

MEASURING AND EVALUATING LEG LENGTH

Leg-length differences can be in the upper leg (femoral) or in the lower leg (tibial).

- Physicians traditionally determine leg length by measuring the distance from the pelvis to the ankle—specifically, the distance from the anterior superior iliac spine to the medial malleolus.
- X rays can be used to measure the length of the legs more accurately.
- It's easy to quickly eyeball and measure upper and lower leg-length differences. Sit the rider with the back flat against a hard-backed chair, feet on the ground. Place a straightedge in front of the anterior (forward) protrusion of the kneecaps—point A in Figure 4-6. If an upper leg-length discrepancy is present, the straightedge will not be level against the knees. When the straightedge is level against the longer leg, the distance to the straightedge from the shorter leg is the upper length discrepancy. Differences of a few millimeters are usually insignificant. Place a straightedge on the superior (top) part of the knee—point B in Figure 4-6. If a lower leg-length discrepancy is present, the straightedge will not be level on the knees. When the straightedge is level against the longer leg, the distance to the straightedge from the shorter leg is the lower length discrepancy. Differences of a few millimeters are usually insignificant.

Figure 4-6

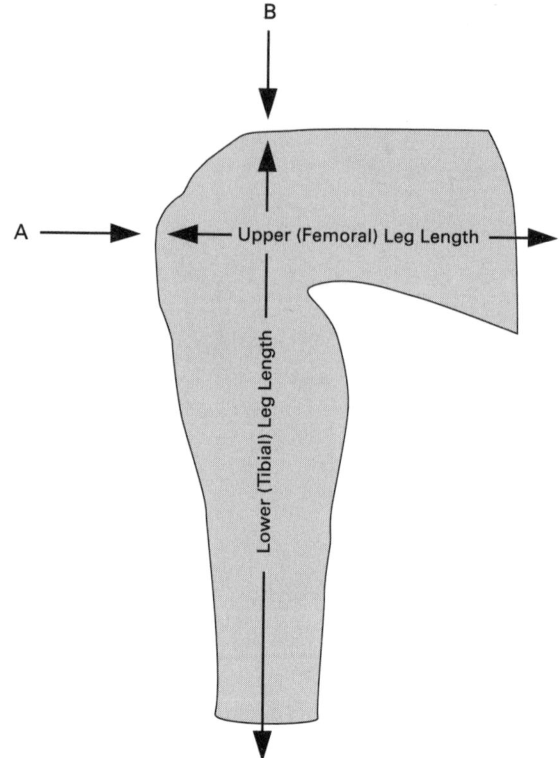

Measuring upper and lower leg lengths

EVALUATING LEG LENGTH BY KNEE ANGLES

Measuring leg length may not reveal the real issue. Some riders with no leg-length difference, for example, have an effective difference when riding because of arthritic changes in the hips or other factors. And some riders have accommodated to their differences with their pedaling styles.

Another approach is to measure the angles of the knees when pedaling. If they are equal, then the legs are effectively the same length. If they are different, the legs are effectively of different lengths, regardless of actual measurements.

The traditional method of measuring knee angles is to have the rider stop pedaling at the bottom of the stroke and measure knee angle with a goniometer: a protractor with long arms.

Many riders change the angle of the knee when they stop pedaling by changing their ankle position. Measuring knee angles with an electronic goniometer while the rider pedals gives more accurate information.

HOW TO CORRECT FOR LEG-LENGTH DISCREPANCY

Set the seat height for the longer leg. Shim the exterior sole or cleat of the shoe on the shorter leg to equalize knee angles.

The body partially adapts to leg-length differences. In general, femoral (upper leg) differences require about one-third correction, tibial (lower leg) differences about one-half. So, for example, a femoral leg length discrepancy of 6 millimeters requires about a 2-millimeter shim. A tibial leg length discrepancy of 6 millimeters requires about a 3-millimeter shim.

Some femoral differences can also be partially accommodated by offsetting the cleat of the shorter leg forward (cycling more on the toes). Small differences are sometimes shimmed with an insole. This often crowds the interior of the shoe and is not ideal. The insole of the shoe of the longer leg is sometimes removed as an easy fix for small differences. Again, a comfortable fit may now not be possible. Different-size shoes to accommodate different thicknesses of insoles are an unusual and rare alternative.

Some practitioners correct leg-length differences with eccentric chainrings, concentrically machined but off-center mounted chainrings, or different-length cranks. I do not endorse these approaches.

Muscle Cramps

Muscle cramps can and do affect almost all riders. What can really be done to help prevent this problem, and what can be done once cramps occur?

WHAT ARE MUSCLE CRAMPS?

Cramps are involuntary muscle contractions or spasms, often sustained and painful.

WHAT CAUSES CRAMPS?

There are probably many causes of cramps. No one is certain why cramps occur in any individual. Though many suggestions have been offered to help prevent cramps, there is probably as much folklore as science in most recommendations.

Some of the more likely causes are these:

- Fluid and electrolyte imbalance. This is probably more of a problem in the local muscle cell area than a reflection of overall body electrolyte imbalance or dehydration. Some of the electrolytes implicated are magnesium, potassium, and calcium.
- Temperature changes—unacclimatized cold or hot weather.
- Low blood sugar.
- Unaccustomed sudden hard exertion or inadequate conditioning.
- Fatigue.

- Accumulation of waste products, such as lactic acid.
- Lack of flexibility.
- Medical problems or diseases (an unusual but possible cause of cramps).

PREVENTION

- Train specifically—if you are a racer and will have surges and jumps in your races, train that way.
- Eat a diet rich in carbohydrates, calcium, potassium, and magnesium.
- Eat during long rides.
- Be adequately hydrated before and during rides and races.
- Allow time for acclimatization if you are traveling.

TREATMENT OF CRAMPS

- Stretch or massage the cramp. You may be able to do this while continuing to ride, or the cramp may force you to stop.
- Apply hot or cold packs. Either may help.

Knees—Introduction

WHAT WE'RE TALKING ABOUT

Knee problems are common in cyclists.

We're talking about overuse injuries—knee problems related to the repeated and constant stresses of riding over time—which are one of the most frequent reasons cyclists seek medical advice.

Some knee problems are the result of sudden injuries related to trauma: a bicycle crash, or the sudden tearing of a cartilage or ligament. Sudden injuries, injuries with significant local swelling (water on the knee), knee clicking, knee instability, and knee collapse are not discussed here. Torn ligaments, torn menisci, and fractures generally require prompt professional medical attention.

Significant local redness or warmth may indicate an infection and requires prompt medical attention. Those with a history of gout or other forms of arthritis are advised to seek medical attention. The different kinds of knee arthritis are not discussed in this book.

With proper positioning, cycling helps many knee problems.

Note: As is the case throughout this book, the topic is discussed for informational purposes, not as a substitute for professional care. Although mild problems may be self-treated, any problem that does not respond within a couple of weeks needs expert advice.

KNEE LOCATION AS A CLUE TO TREATMENT

Knee complaints can usually be identified as being in the front (anterior), inside (medial), outside (lateral), or back (posterior) of the knee. Internal (within) derangements of the knee are mostly left out of this book—they generally require orthopedic consultation.

Even without understanding the root of the problem, knowing where the knee hurts makes it possible to recommend certain bicycle-position changes.

Bicycle Position Adjustment for Knee Pain

The basic position considerations are seat position and foot position.

The seat may be

- Too low or too high.
- Too far forward or too far back.

The feet may be

- Too far apart or too close together.
- Too toed in or toed out.
- Too far forward or too far back in relationship to the pedal axle.

When the problem is the distance between the feet, correction may be made by

- Changing the cleat position.
- Using a different length of bottom bracket axle.
- Using cranks with a different offset.
- Using a shim between the pedal axle and the crank.

Foot rotation may be a factor:

- Pedal flotation allows the foot to rotate on the bicycle pedal. This freedom of motion has helped many riders for whom the fixed-cleat position has contributed to knee strain.
- Too much float may also be harmful; a limitation of flotation may allow some overuse injuries to improve.

Table 4-1

Knee Pain Causes and Diagnosis

Location	Causes	Solutions
Front of knee (Anterior)	Seat too low	Raise seat
	Seat too forward	Move seat back
	Climbing too much	Reduce climbing
	Big gears, low r.p.m.	Spin more
	Cranks too long	Shorten cranks
Inside of knee (Medial)	Cleats — toes point out	Modify cleat position — toe in
		Consider floating pedals
	Floating pedals	Limit float to 5 degrees
	Exiting clipless pedals	Lower tension
	Feet too far apart	Modify cleat position — closer
		Shorten bottom bracket axle
		Use cranks with less offset
Outside of knee (Lateral)	Cleats — toes point in	Modify cleat — toe out
		Consider floating pedals
	Floating pedals	Limit float to 5 degrees
	Feet too close	Modify cleat position — apart
		Longer bottom bracket axle
		Use cranks with more offset
		Shim pedal on crank 2 millimeters
Back of knee (Posterior)	Saddle too high	Lower saddle
	Saddle too far back	Move saddle forward
	Floating pedals	Limit float to 5 degrees

ANATOMY OF THE KNEE

The major anatomical landmarks of the knee are shown in Figures 4-7 and 4-8.

Figure 4-7

Front view of the knee (patella and quadriceps removed)

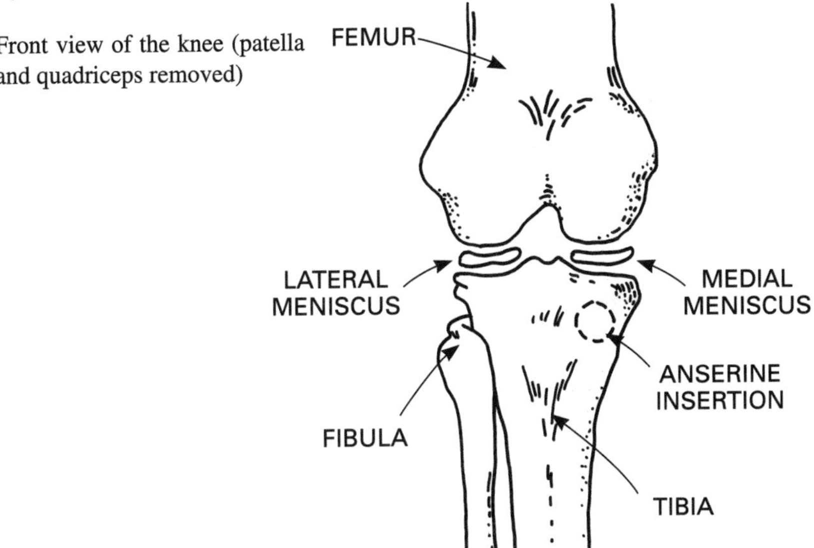

Figure 4-8

Side view of the knee

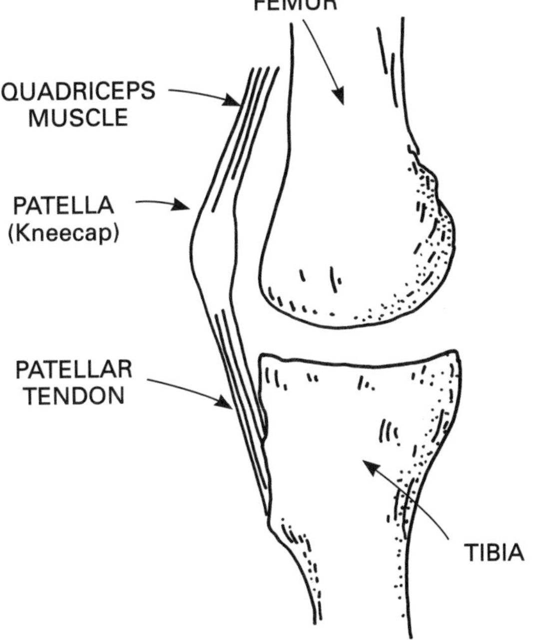

Chondromalacia Patellae (Front of the Knee—Anterior)

WHAT WE'RE TALKING ABOUT

The kneecap, or patella, is in front of the knee. It glides over the end of the thigh bone, or femur. Sometimes the underside surface of the kneecap is roughened, or softened, and instead of gliding smoothly it rubs roughly over the end of the thigh bone. This problem is sometimes called patellofemoral dysfunction, or patellofemoral syndrome, because of the anatomic location of this problem.

A grating sensation at the front of the knee, pain going down stairs, and a general ache are frequent features. Stiffness after prolonged seating (moviegoer's stiffness) is common.

Figure 4-9

Front-of-the-knee tenderness. Tenderness here is usually due to chondromalacia or arthritis.

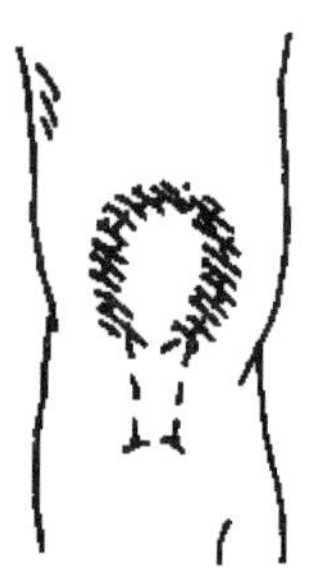

CAUSES

The kneecap, or patella, is not flat on its underside but has a ridge. As the knee bends, this ridge follows a path along the surface of the thigh bone, or femur.

Excessive force pushing the kneecap onto the surface of the end of the thigh bone creates excessive stress—called loading or shearing force—on the underside of the kneecap and may result in its surface becoming roughened.

Some individuals are genetically predisposed to a rough kneecap. A muscle or posture imbalance may cause the kneecap to stray from its ideal path over the surface of the femur. When not gliding over its ideal path, the patella is subject to increased forces and becomes roughened. A relative weakness of the inside or medial quadriceps muscles is often responsible. A wide pelvis and "knock-knees" may make the condition more likely.

Some of the bicycling causes of excessive loading or shearing forces are hill climbing and big-gear time trialing. Weight training, running, squatting, kneeling, and climbing also place increased pressure on the patellar-femoral surface.

This tends to be an early season injury.

TREATMENTS

On the Bicycle

Bicycling done correctly often helps this problem. Many runners suffer from chondromalacia, and bicycle riding is often suggested for therapy. A roughened kneecap will often smooth out over time if offending activities are stopped.

A relatively high-in-the-saddle position helps—make sure your knee is not bent more than 25 degrees from horizontal when your foot is at the bottom of your stroke. Sit farther back in the saddle. Spin rather than use big gears—maintain a cadence of 85 r.p.m. or more. Avoid hills, especially long climbs. Stand more when climbing. Avoid long cranks.

If pain is due to a tracking problem, rather than a load problem, pedals allowing some free rotation may help.

Off the Bicycle

Weight-lifting machines usually increase the load or shearing forces of the patella on the femur. Exercises that bend the knee more than 90 degrees place tremendously increased loads on those surfaces and may worsen your problem. Squats, leg presses, and leg extensions all place increased loads on the patellofemoral surface.

Avoid squatting, kneeling, going walking, or running down stairs or hills. Avoid running. Above all, avoid running down hills.

Medical Treatment

R.I.C.E. Discussed on page 167.

Strengthening. Strengthening the medial quadriceps may help. You are looking for exercises that involve only the last part of straightening your leg. Remember, be cautious about strength training when you are injured. Use strength training primarily to prevent reinjury. Machines that limit the bend in your knee to 15 to 20 degrees from straight out, and then allow you to complete the last 15 to 20 degrees of extension, are helpful. You might try placing a couple of pillows under your knee while lying down. With weight around your ankle, lift and straighten your knee, hold for a couple of seconds, then relax. Repeat up to 100 times. Athletes may use weights up to about one quarter of body weight. Elite cyclists may have difficulty placing enough weight on their ankle to make this exercise worthwhile.

Step-ups to a height of one step may be helpful. With only your body weight at first, face a 8- to 10-inch step, and place the foot of your affected leg on the step. Raise yourself up. Lower yourself. Repeat fifteen to twenty times. As you develop balance and understand the exercise you may hold weights in your hands or place a barbell on your back. Elite cyclists may lift up to their body weight in barbell load.

Isometric exercises with the leg outstretched and no change in position during the exercise may be helpful. Since this exercise can be performed in any position—standing, sitting, or lying—it's easy to perform hundreds of 20- to 30-second repetitions daily.

Stretching. Quadriceps exercises are particularly useful. See page 150.

NSAIDs. Discussed on page 161.

Orthotics. If excessive foot pronation results in inside-of-the-kneecap discomfort, orthotics or medial wedges may help.

Cortisone. Not used in this location.

Surgery. The treatment of last resort. The underside of the roughed kneecap may be smoothed. If the gliding path of the kneecap is incorrect, repositioning tendons may be tried. This is a drastic step.

Patellar Tendonitis (Front of the Knee—Anterior)

WHAT WE'RE TALKING ABOUT

The patellar tendon attaches the bottom of the patella—or kneecap—to the tibial tubercle, a prominence on the front top of the shin bone.

As with other tendons, inflammation or irritation of this tendon results in tendonitis. This type of tendonitis may take a relatively long time to resolve with continued riding.

A specific variant of this problem—Osgood-Schlatter's disease—is found mostly in adolescent boys. In this case, pain occurs at the point where the patella tendon attaches to the shin bone.

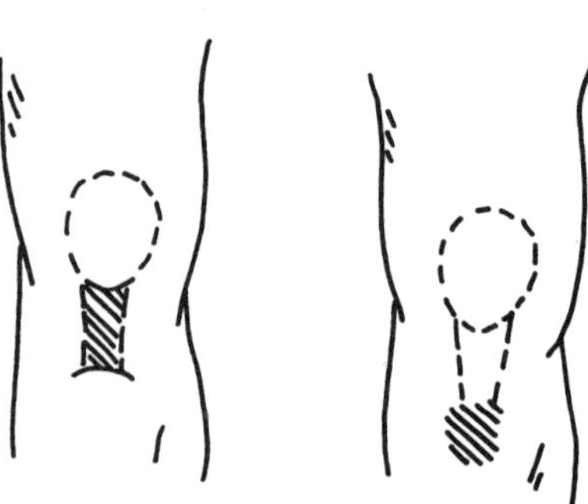

Figure 4-10

Front-of-the-knee tenderness. Tenderness in the shaded area at left is usually due to patellar tendonitis. Tenderness in the shaded area at right is usually due to Osgood-Schlatter's disease.

CAUSES

Tendonitis in this area from repetitive bicycling stress may follow a one-time injury to this area or may result from poor bike fit. Low saddle, forward position, big gears, and long hills all contribute to this problem. Some people's anatomy predisposes them to this condition.

In Osgood-Schlatter's disease, growth of the bones during the growth spurt results in a pulling at the point where the patellar tendon meets the tibial tubercle—the forward top prominence of the shin bone.

Tenderness at the kneecap's lower edge is occasionally due to a stress fracture.

TREATMENTS

On the Bicycle

A relatively high-in-the-saddle position helps—make sure your knee is not bent more than 25 degrees from horizontal when your foot is at the bottom of your stroke. Sit farther back in the saddle. Spin rather than use big gears—maintain a cadence of 85 r.p.m. or more. Avoid hills, especially long climbs. Avoid long cranks. Limit flotation to 5 degrees.

Off the Bicycle

Same as for chondromalacia, above. Jumping sports are particularly associated with patellar tendonitis.

Medical Treatment

See chondromalacia patellae, above.

R.I.C.E. May be helpful; discussed on page 167.

Stretching. Discussed on page 150.

Orthotics. Can be helpful.

NSAIDs. Discussed on page 161.

Cortisone. Not used in this location.

Surgery. Not used in this location.

Quadriceps Tendonitis (Front of the Knee—Anterior)

WHAT WE'RE TALKING ABOUT

The quadriceps tendons attach the ends of the quadriceps muscles to either the upper pole of the patella—the kneecap—or the shin bone. As with other tendons, inflammation or irritation in this area results in tendonitis. This type of tendonitis may take a relatively long time to resolve with continued riding.

CAUSES

Tendonitis in this area from repetitive bicycling stress may follow a one-time injury to this area or may result from poor bike fit. Low saddle, forward position, big gears, and long hills all contribute to this problem.

TREATMENT

Same as for patellar tendonitis and chondromalacia, above, unless the medial (inside) quadriceps muscle is involved, in which case terminal extension exercises are to be avoided as well.

Pre-Patellar Bursitis (Front of the Knee—Anterior)

WHAT WE'RE TALKING ABOUT

Swelling and perhaps some discomfort over the lower kneecap and patellar tendon caused by a swelling of the covering envelope, or bursa. If this area is red, warm, or tender, see a physician to make sure it is not infected.

CAUSES

Overuse irritation from frequent prolonged kneeling. Commonly seen in carpet layers and floor-scrubbers—"housemaid's knee." Continued irritation from an initial injury, such as a fall, occurs in cyclists.

TREATMENT

Off the Bicycle

Avoid kneeling. Use knee pads if kneeling must be continued. Otherwise, treatment is the same as for patellar tendonitis and chondromalacia, above.

Medical Treatment

NSAIDs. Discussed on page 161.

Cortisone. Fluid drainage and cortisone treatment has a fair success rate.

Surgery. May be required to remove a chronically inflamed bursa.

Arthritis (Front of the Knee—Anterior)

WHAT WE'RE TALKING ABOUT

Many forms of knee arthritis exist. The most common, osteoarthritis (degenerative joint disease), occurs as we age. It is simply the result of wear and tear on the joint. Pain or ache is felt in the front of the knee or throughout the knee.

CAUSES

Wear and tear from aging. The additional knee stress brought about by obesity, pushing big gears, or climbing may also contribute.

TREATMENT

Same as for chondromalacia, above.

NSAIDs. A mainstay of treatment, discussed on page 161.

Cortisone. Occasionally used.

Surgery. Used in the most severe cases. It may include total knee replacement.

Anserine Tendonitis (Inside of the Knee—Medial)

WHAT WE'RE TALKING ABOUT

The anserine tendon attaches at the upper inner aspect of the shin bone. It is really the coming together of three muscles: semitendinosus, gracilis, and sartorius. This tendon, or its bursa underneath, becomes irritated and inflamed.

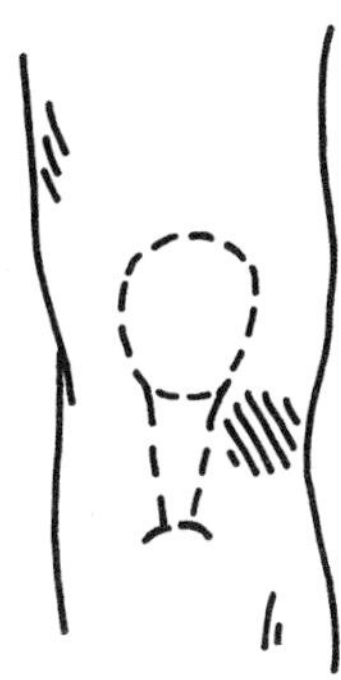

Figure 4-11

Inside-of-the-knee tenderness (right knee). Tenderness here is often due to anserine tendonitis.

CAUSES OF ANSERINE TENDONITIS

Increased pressure on the inside of the knee. Extra force is put on this area by having your toes pointed outward or your knees too far apart when cycling. Exiting clipless pedals stresses the ligaments and tendons at the inside of the knee. Occasionally, improper saddle position is a factor.

Some people's anatomy predisposes them to this condition—turned-in shin bones, pronation, and bowed legs.

TREATMENTS

On the Bicycle

If you use fixed cleats, adjust them so that the toes point a little more inward. If you use floating pedals, limit flotation to 5 degrees. Reduce the tension of your clipless pedals to allow you to exit them more easily. Reduce the distance between your feet by (1) positioning your cleat so that your foot is closer to the crank, (2) using a narrower bottom bracket axle, or (3) using cranks with less offset. Use a proper saddle position and spin over 85 r.p.m. Reduce mileage.

Off the Bicycle

Avoid running on inclines, especially when the affected leg is on the uphill side. Roller blading and skiing may make this problem worse.

Medical Treatment

R.I.C.E. Useful, discussed on page 167.

Stretching. An important therapy.

NSAIDs. Useful, discussed on page 161.

Orthotics. May help this problem.

Cortisone. Used for this problem.

Surgery. Rarely used for this problem and is a last resort.

Plica—Patellofemoral Ligament (Inside of the Knee—Medial)

WHAT WE'RE TALKING ABOUT

A plica is a thickened fibrous band of tissue. Either the medial patellofemoral ligament—a ligament between the kneecap and the thigh bone, on the inside of the knee—gets irritated and inflamed, or a fold within the knee develops a similar problem.

This causes pain either on the inside (medial) aspect of the knee or within the knee itself. Pain frequently occurs within a reproducible range of motion—once on the downstroke, once on the upstroke. A torn medial meniscus or cartilage may also produce similar symptoms. Often, only surgery will distinguish the true diagnosis.

If you have locking or swelling of your knee, consult an orthopedist or sports medicine physician.

CAUSES

Increased pressure on the inside of the knee is related to the problem. Extra force is caused by having your toes pointed outward or your knees too far apart when cycling. Occasionally, improper saddle position is a factor. Some people's anatomy tends to predispose them to this condition—those with turned-in shin bones, pronation, and bowed legs.

TREATMENTS

On the Bicycle

If you use fixed cleats, adjust them so that the toes point a little more inward. If you use floating pedals, limit flotation to 5 degrees. Reduce the distance between your feet by (1) positioning your cleat so that your foot is closer to the crank, (2) using a narrower bottom bracket axle, or (3) using cranks with less offset. Use a proper saddle position and spin over 85 r.p.m. Reduce mileage.

Off the Bicycle

Cyclists have this problem as often as other athletes. Running, skiing, and in-line skating make the problem worse.

Medical Treatment

R.I.C.E. Discussed on page 167.

Stretching. May help.

NSAIDs. Discussed on page 161.

Orthotics. May help this problem.

Cortisone. Not used for this problem.

Surgery. Used for this problem. Surgery may be necessary to correctly differentiate between medial plica, medial patellofemoral ligament, and medial meniscal problems. Knee locking and repeated knee swelling may indicate the need for surgery.

Iliotibial Band Syndrome (Outside of Knee—Lateral)

WHAT WE'RE TALKING ABOUT

The iliotibial band (ITB) is a fibrous band of tissue running along the outside of the knee. It rubs over the outside surface of the knee, especially when the knee is bent about 30 degrees. It is commonly inflamed, causing pain in this area.

Figure 4-12

Outside-of-the-knee tenderness—right knee. Tenderness here is often due to iliotibial band tendonitis.

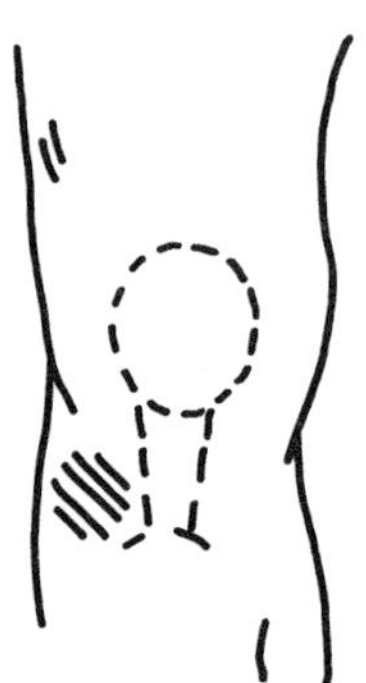

CAUSES OF ILIOTIBIAL BAND SYNDROME

Excessive stretch on this area, from too much pull on the outside of the knee, is the most common cause. Maladjusted cleat position, with the toes pointing in, is the most frequent cause of this pulling. A narrow bottom bracket or cranks with little offset may be associated with ITB syndrome. Low saddle height and excessive forces due to big gears and hills are contributing factors. Sometimes iliotibial band syndrome develops after a fall and a bruise to this area. Some people's anatomy predisposes them to this condition, especially those with a wide pelvis. Tight gluteal muscles can be a contributing factor.

TREATMENTS

On the Bicycle

Readjust your cleats to allow your toes to point out a little more. Limit flotation to 5 degrees. Increase the distance between your feet by (1) positioning your cleats so that your foot is farther from the crank, (2) inserting a 2-millimeter spacer between the pedal and the crank, (3) using a wider bottom bracket, or (4) using cranks with more offset. Reduce hill work. A floating pedal system may help. Make sure your saddle height is not too low or too high, and not too far back.

Off the Bicycle

Avoid running, especially on canted surfaces where the affected leg is uphill from the unaffected one.

Medical Treatment

R.I.C.E. Discussed on page 167.

Strengthening. Side kicks and slide board exercises may help or worsen this problem.

Stretching. Specific stretches discussed and shown on page 150 are useful.

Orthotics. Can help this problem.

NSAIDs. Discussed on page 161.

Cortisone. Can be used in this location if other methods fail.

Surgery. A last resort.

Tight Hamstrings (Back of the Knee—Posterior)

WHAT WE'RE TALKING ABOUT

The muscles in the back of the thigh are known as the hamstrings. Tightness in this area is a common cause of pain behind the knee.

CAUSES

High seat position and sitting too far back in the saddle are contributing factors. Dropping the heel when climbing, and pushing big gears, worsen the problem. Lack of flexibility is usually present. Improper cleat position can be a factor in fixed-pedal systems. Sometimes excessive pedal float can be related to this problem because the hamstrings help stabilize the leg when pedaling. Relative weakness of the hamstrings compared with the strength of the quads can be a contributing factor.

TREATMENTS

On the Bicycle

Sit farther forward in the saddle. Avoid a high saddle position. Avoid dropping your heels when pushing a big gear or climbing. Use pedals that limit your float to less than 5 degrees.

Medical Treatment

R.I.C.E. Useful; discussed on page 167.

Strengthening. Tight hamstrings are often weak hamstrings. Strengthening exercises are useful.

Stretching. The most important therapy.

NSAIDs. Discussed on page 161.

Orthotics. Rarely help this problem.

Cortisone. Not used for this problem.

Surgery. Rarely used for this problem and is a last resort.

Baker's Cyst (Back of the Knee—Posterior)

WHAT WE'RE TALKING ABOUT

Baker's cyst is found behind the knee. It is a swelling of a sac that has its origins within the knee, or of a bursa associated with a muscle behind the knee. It is an occasional cause of pain behind the knee. If the cyst ruptures, it can cause calf pain that may mimic the pain of a blood clot.

CAUSES

The cause is a weakness in the tissues. When associated with a sac that has its origins within the knee, it often indicates a more serious problem within the knee.

TREATMENTS

On the Bicycle

Sit farther forward in the saddle. Avoid a high saddle position. Avoid dropping your heels when pushing a big gear or climbing.

Medical Treatment

R.I.C.E. Discussed on page 167.

Stretching. Probably not helpful.

NSAIDs. Discussed on page 161.

Orthotics. Not helpful with this problem.

Cortisone. Not used for this problem.

Surgery. Frequently helpful in removing the cyst and curing the problem. It may also be helpful in correcting any internal knee problems related to a Baker's cyst.

Tibialis Anterior Tendonitis

WHAT WE'RE TALKING ABOUT

Inflammation of the shin muscles. "Shin splints" or anterior lower leg pain is much more common in runners.

CAUSES

Excessive tendon strain on the upstroke, especially when the foot is dorsiflexed (bent upward).

TREATMENT

On the Bicycle

Avoid a forceful pull up. Occasionally a high saddle contributes to the problem; lowering the saddle may help.

Off the Bicycle

Avoid running, especially on hills.

Medical Treatment

R.I.C.E. Discussed on page 167.

NSAIDs. Discussed on page 161.

Achilles Tendonitis

WHAT WE'RE TALKING ABOUT

Tendonitis, or inflammation of the Achilles tendon: the giant tendon at the bottom of the back of your leg. A different problem in this area is bursitis—see the next article below. For pain on the bottom of the heel, see "Heel Pain Syndrome—Plantar Fasciitis," page 231.

Problems in this area are not unusual in cyclists, but they occur less frequently than knee overuse problems.

CAUSES

Excessive stretch from unaccustomed activity usually causes the problem. This most often results from a new shoe or cleat, especially when the next consequence is that the extension of your leg has been increased. For example, if you are used to the Shimano clipless system and change to Speedplay, the shoe–pedal distance is reduced. This means you'll need to lower your seat. If you don't, excess stretch occurs, and you are at risk for Achilles tendonitis.

Somewhat paradoxically, a seat that is too low can also cause a problem. In an attempt to get more power, the rider may drop the back of the foot on the downstroke, placing excessive and repeated stretch on the Achilles tendon. If you have unequal leg lengths, the shorter leg is more likely to have an Achilles tendon problem. A cleat too far forward or positioned so that the foot is toed in can occasionally cause this problem. Soft or flexible soles may contribute to the condition. Cold, wet-weather riding, when the back of the sock gets wet and cold, may cause the problem.

TREATMENT

On the Bicycle

Ride if you are pain free. Hills are usually harder on the Achilles tendon, so reduce hill mileage. Reduce the stretch on your Achilles tendon. For most riders, this means lowering the saddle a few millimeters.

Off the Bicycle

If this injury is associated with other activity, that activity may need to be modified. For example, if you've switched to a lower heel on your walking shoe, a heel pad or lift may help.

Medical Treatment

R.I.C.E. Rest and hot or cold compresses may be helpful.

Stretching. Important once your problem improves, not while it's painful.

Orthotics. Can help this problem.

NSAIDs. May be helpful.

Cortisone. Never. Don't get a cortisone injection here—it weakens the tendon and may cause rupture.

Surgery. A last resort.

Achilles Bursitis

WHAT WE'RE TALKING ABOUT

The medical name is posterior calcaneal bursitis, commonly called a pump bump.

CAUSE

The heel counter (back part) of an offending shoe irritates the bursa.

TREATMENT

Avoid the offending shoe, or cut out the offending heel counter.

Medical Treatment

R.I.C.E. Hot or cold compresses may be helpful.

NSAIDs. May be helpful.

Cortisone. Occasionally helpful. Don't get a cortisone injection if the problem is tendonitis—it weakens the tendon and may cause rupture.

Surgery. A last resort.

Ankle Sprain

WHAT WE'RE TALKING ABOUT

Ankle sprain is the stretching or tearing of ligament fibers that support either the outside or the inside of the ankle. If there is not much swelling or tenderness over the bones of your ankle, if you can walk normally, and if there is no blood bruising of the skin, you may try treatment on your own. If you have swelling, if you have tenderness over the bones of your ankle, if you can't bear weight on your ankle, if you have blood bruising of the skin, or if it's the inside of your ankle that hurts, consult a physician.

CAUSES

Most sprains result from an inward twisting motion of the foot, and most of the time the outside of the ankle is sprained. Occasionally it's the inside that has the problem. The cause is not usually cycling-related per se. Sprains usually happen when you're a little klutzy, just like they happen to non-riders. Cleats that allow too much float may aggravate ankle sprains.

CLASSIFICATION OF ANKLE SPRAIN

Ankle sprains are graded into three groups. Grade one sprains are the least severe; grade three are the most severe.

- *Grade one* sprains involve tearing of less than 20% of the ligament fibers. They have minimal swelling, and you are able to bear your weight on your injury. There is no blood bruising of the skin.
- *Grade two* sprains involve tearing of 20% to 70% of the ligament fibers. They have moderate swelling, and walking is difficult. Blood bruising of the skin is usually present.
- *Grade three* sprains involve tearing more than 70% of the ligament fibers. Swelling is at least moderate. Walking is impossible. Blood bruising of the skin is present. (A complete rupture is 100% tearing of the ligament fibers.)

TREATMENT

All sprains are treated initially with R.I.C.E.—rest, ice, compression, and elevation. All are treated with anti-inflammatory and pain medicines as needed. Get a doctor's care for all but the least severe sprains; an X ray is usually needed to make sure no fracture is present. Broken ankles are not discussed in this book.

Grade one sprains may be treated with a weight-bearing brace or strapping for a couple of weeks. Ace wraps usually don't provide much support; a Conform bandage or athletic strapping provides better support.

Grade two sprains are treated in the same way as grade one sprains. Additional support may be needed longer. A weight-bearing shoe may be needed for a few weeks. Crutches are usually used. An Aircast™ ankle brace or other support may be helpful. Flexion-extension exercises are begun after forty-eight hours. Full-ankle range of motion exercises are begun a couple of weeks after the injury.

Grade three sprains may need an Aircast™ or a traditional cast for several weeks. Surgery may be required.

LONG-TERM COMPLICATIONS

All sprains make you a little less coordinated, and all are associated with frequent re-injury. Once you've sprained your ankle, and some of the ligament fibers are torn, some of the nerve fibers may be stretched too. You don't get the proper feedback from your foot. It is sometimes hard to know exactly where your foot is! Prevent further reinjury by being aware of this problem and by being careful.

Inadequate rest can delay healing and cause a relatively minor sprain to persist longer than it would otherwise. Persistent swelling following an ankle sprain is common. Occasionally the initial injury combined with the repeated stress of riding causes a tendonitis.

If you have sprained your ankle, have proper support, and find that it hurts more after riding, it is sensible to back off riding until your injury is healed. Severe sprains may result in long-term ankle weakness and instability. They may require surgery.

Heel Pain Syndrome—Plantar Fasciitis

WHAT WE'RE TALKING ABOUT

Pain on the bottom of the heel. For pain on the back of the heel, see "Achilles Tendonitis," page 228.

The plantar fascia is a fibrous band in the foot's arch that runs from the toes to the heel. It helps support the arch and prevent it from collapsing. Inflammation of this band—plantar fasciitis—is the usual problem.

Sometimes a bone spur, or pointed growth of bone, develops where the foot ligaments attach to the heel bone, or calcaneus.

CAUSES

Inflammation occurs where the plantar fascia attaches to the heel as a result of excessive repetitive stretch from chronic foot strain. Excessive pronation and a low-arched or a high-arched foot are common causes. The immediate cause of this problem is not often related to cycling. But many things cyclists do—running and weight lifting—are associated with the problem. It also may be related to non-cycling shoes that are too stiff-soled, being overweight, hiking, or carrying heavy loads.

An X ray may or may not show a spur. Usually the spur is indication of a long-term problem—it is not itself the cause of the pain.

TREATMENT

Stretch! Facing a wall, with your foot planted about 3 feet from the wall, lean against the wall with your leg straight. Repeat with your knee bent. You should feel a pull in your calf. Read "Stretching" in the chapter "Physical Therapy," page 164. Increasing the flexibility of your Achilles tendon reduces the need for this area to stretch and reduces strain on the plantar fascia.

Foot exercises may be helpful. Here are two to try:

1. Walk on the outsides of your bare feet for ten minutes twice a day.
2. With your foot bare, use your toes to grab hold of and lift up a face cloth. Hold for a count of five. Let go. Build up to 20 times twice a day.

- A heel pad or waffle support, also known as a Tuli's cup, may help.
- Icing ten minutes twice a day may help.
- Anti-inflammatory medicines may help.
- Local steroid injection has a fair success rate.
- An orthotic may help.

Foot or Toe Numbness—Hot and Cold Foot

WHAT WE'RE TALKING ABOUT

Pain, burning, or numbness in the ball of the foot or the toes. In cool weather, the foot may be cold.

CAUSES

Pain, burning, or numbness is almost always caused by pressure around the foot. Old-style cleats with toe straps that are too tight, shoes that are too tight, or shoe straps cinched too tightly are the usual causes. Occasionally high mileage and an improperly positioned cleat contribute to the problem. Sometimes the cause is arthritis or an unusual medical condition. In cool weather, cold feet may result from compression of the foot and the resulting decrease in blood circulation.

TREATMENT

For pain, burning, or numbness, the solution is to relieve the pressure. Loosen your toe straps, loosen your shoes, buy wider or larger shoes. When you stop for lunch or take a rest stop—even if only for a few minutes—take off your shoes and wiggle your toes.

Occasionally the problem relates to cleat position. Usually the cleat needs to be placed farther back, although solutions differ. Do whatever allows the foot more room in the shoe. An irregularity of the sole (occasionally a manufacturing defect) may press on the ball of your foot. Look for cleat bolts that are pushing through the sole, causing it to be uneven. Too much or too little cleat/shoe contact may contribute to the problem.

Orthotics, which can spread the pressure, may help.

Occasionally the problem relates to a swollen nerve: a Morton's neuroma.

Local cortisone injection, orthotics, or surgical removal of the neuroma are options. If your problem persists, see your doctor.

For cold feet, relieve the pressure. Consider wider or larger shoes that allow room for thermal socks, or use shoe covers.

Head, Ears, Eyes, Nose, and Mouth

Head Injury

It is possible to die while riding a bicycle. Head injury is the most likely cause. This chapter could also be titled "Wear a Helmet—Here's Why!"

WHAT WE'RE TALKING ABOUT

- About 1,000 bicycling deaths each year are caused by head injuries.
- About 80% of all cycling deaths result from head injuries.
- 60% to 70% of all serious bicycle injuries involve head trauma.
- 50% of head-injury deaths occur in adults, 50% in children and adolescents.
- The head injury risk is reduced 85% to 95% by use of a helmet.

WHEN TO WEAR A HELMET

- Always wear a helmet.
- Wear a CPSC-, Snell-, or ANSI-approved and -tested helmet.
- Wear a helmet for high-risk rides—mountain biking, criteriums, and track races.
- Wear a helmet for moderate-risk rides—road races, time trials, group rides.
- Wear a helmet for low-risk rides—commuting, warming up for races.
- Wear a helmet for very low-risk rides—going a half block to the store, checking bike fit, riding two blocks to your friend's house.
- Encourage your friends to wear a helmet. "Friends don't let friends ride without a helmet."
- Dismiss petty excuses. *Heat* is not an issue. Helmets have no significant effect in overheating riders on hot days. *Aerodynamics* is improved in comparison with riding bare-headed. *Weight* is of trifling significance; helmets weigh about half a pound. *Cost* is a non-issue. Cost is a fraction of a single emergency room visit, about the same as a routine doctor's office visit. *Fashion* is not an excuse. Modern helmets look "cool."
- Always wear a helmet!

HELMET FIT

To be effective, a helmet must be properly fitted. It needs to be the right size and worn covering the forehead, and the straps must be snug.

BROKEN HELMET?

It did its job. Get another one before you ride again. Many helmet manufacturers will replace broken helmets free or at nominal cost. If you crash on your helmet, you should replace it even if you see no visible defect. The helmet may be weakened. Never ride with a helmet that has been involved in a previous accident.

I remember riding with a guy who had had a head injury and wasn't wearing a helmet. I asked him how he injured his head. "I broke my helmet last week in a crash—I crashed again, and this time I hit my head, instead of my helmet, when I fell," he answered!

CONCUSSION

Concussion is an injury to the brain, usually related to a blow to the head. The brain doesn't work right for a while. You may be knocked out or have memory loss.

Is Concussion Serious?

Any concussion is potentially dangerous. The longer a person is unconscious, or the longer the memory loss, the worse the concussion. Serious concussion can occur even if there is not a loss of consciousness, a cut, or a bump on the head. Concussion can result in permanent brain damage and death.

Emergency Room—Doctor Visit?

Always—if you've had any memory loss or loss of consciousness.

Seek Medical Attention If Any of the Following Develop:

- Loss of consciousness
- Convulsions (seizures)
- Memory loss
- Confusion
- Restlessness, irritability
- Garbled speech
- Vomiting more than once
- Unusual sleepiness or decreasing alertness
- Pupils of different sizes
- Trouble using arms or legs
- Fever
- Bleeding from the nose or ears

- Headaches that don't ease up, especially those not directly underneath the area struck

Pain Medicine?

Acetaminophen (Tylenol) is OK. Do not use narcotics, which might have side effects that can be confused with concussion, or anti-inflammatories—such as aspirin, ibuprofen, or naproxen—which might increase a bleeding problem related to the injury.

Headache

Some cyclists experience headache during or after rides because of tightness in the neck muscles. Time trialists often experience this problem related to holding the head in a craned position. Mountain bikers may experience this problem because of jarring. Treatment for this problem is described in "Neck Pain," page 188.

Exertional headache may also be a variant of migraine, caused by a spasm in a blood vessel rather than by muscle contraction.

Anti-inflammatory medication—such as over-the-counter aspirin, ibuprofen, or naproxen—may help either preventively or after the fact. Preventive treatment with a variety of other prescription medications is also available. Some of these medications worsen athletic performance. Work with your physician to find the best alternative if prescription medication is necessary.

Earaches

These may be related to riding, though the precise cause isn't known. Earache that persists after riding may be due to the usual other medical causes: swollen lymph glands, dental problems, sinus or ear infection.

A pressure equalization problem in the eustachian tube may be a factor in some earaches. This may be due to allergy, irritants, or unknown factors. Over-the-counter decongestants and antihistamines sometimes help. Prescription medication can provide other options.

Sometimes the problem is related to wind or to cold weather. Cotton in the ear canals is an inexpensive solution for many, but avoid using so much that it interferes with hearing. In cold weather a headband or hat worn under the helmet may help. Actually, they may help in warm weather too—it's just that you'll look weird.

Eye Problems

RED EYES

What We're Talking About

Red or pink eyes whose blood vessels are conspicuous. Irritated eyes. Scratchy eyes.

Causes

Irritants to the eyes. Pollution. Dust. Sweat. Bugs. Allergies to pollens. Wind—especially for contact lens wearers.

Treatment

Protect your eyes with eyewear. Wraparound clear glasses or sunglasses provide the best protection. If you normally wear glasses, you may find oversized lenses more helpful at keeping out wind and irritants than regular or small lenses.

EYEWEAR FEATURES TO LOOK FOR

- *UV protection.* Eye problems such as cataracts and pinguecula—thickening of the inner white corner of the eye—have been linked to ultraviolet light. You are looking for at least 85% UV block, if not 100%.
- *Shatterproof.* "Unbreakable lenses." Polycarbonate provides fantastic impact resistance with only slightly less optical quality than glass.
- *Light reduction.* Clear lenses are fine for cloudy days, but if you live in California or Arizona, your eyes will be a lot more comfortable with sunglasses.

Cool compresses to the eyes can be very soothing. Over-the-counter eye decongestants such as Visine or Murine can help, but if your problem persists, don't abuse the drops—get at the cause.

Contact lens wearers and those whose eyes are dry for other reasons may find a commercial tear or wetting solution helpful.

BUG IN THE EYE

Usually natural tearing will wash the bug to the inside lower corner of your eye. Wiping the corner gently usually rubs it away. Dabbing a corner of moist tissue paper may draw the bug out. Don't rub the cornea, the front, seeing part of your eye.

If tearing doesn't bring the bug to the lower inside corner of your eye, it may be trapped under the upper lid. Carefully dabbing it at this location will usually stick it to the tissue and remove it. Don't dab over the cornea.

The bug may feel as if it's still there if the cornea has become scratched.

If your eye is in spasm and shut, if you can't see properly, if you get a persistent scratchy feeling every time you blink, if pain persists a couple of hours, or if you are not sure, see a doctor.

Runny or Congested Nose

A very common riding situation. Watch any group of riders, and you'll see plenty of them block one nostril with a finger, blow snot out onto the street, then block the other nostril and blow out more.

The nose does "run" more during cycling, sometimes because of allergy or irritants in the air, usually because blood supply to the nose increases and so the nose runs more. Also, the eyes tear more during riding, and the tears flow down through the tear ducts into the nose, causing more secretions to be present.

Some riders use over-the-counter decongestants, antihistamines, or a combination of both to relieve symptoms. The side effects of these medicines are usually not worth the minimum relief they provide most riders. Well-brought-up polite riders discreetly take a tissue from their back pocket and clear their nose at traffic lights or other stops. Most of us get over that and finger-blow while riding—although civility demands that you avoid blowing directly onto other riders. Some move a little to the side, some to the back of the peloton. Still others warn, "Nose blow!"

Ammonia Smell

After long hard workouts, riders sometimes complain of an ammonia smell. It may be due to a product of protein metabolism. Read the chapter "Energy Sources at Various Exercise Levels," beginning on page 16.

Dental Caries

Many riders use energy gels, energy bars, and carbohydrates in solution to help spare, maintain, or increase glycogen stores. The simple sugars in these products have been associated with an increase in cavities, or dental caries.

Lungs and Heart

Dyspnea—Not Enough Air!

The feeling that one can't get enough air is a common medical problem. It occurs in cyclists both in the presence and absence of disease.

WHAT WE'RE TALKING ABOUT

Air hunger—the sensation that there's not enough air. The perception that the lungs can't breath effectively. There's often a feeling of apprehension or anxiety that one can't breathe.

Breathing is controlled by the nervous system in response to varied stimuli. Breathing rates can increase appropriately according to increased metabolic demands during exercise, but they can also increase without metabolic demands, for example, as a result of anxiety or fear.

Normally, individuals are not specifically aware of the act of breathing. With mild exertion, breathing rates may increase and a person may become more conscious of breathing, but discomfort is not felt. With heavy exertion, breathing may become unpleasant, but the individual is aware that this will be transitory and that it is appropriate for the level of exercise.

By contrast, dyspnea is the *abnormally uncomfortable awareness of breathing.*

Dyspnea relates to a change in the aerobic system's capabilities rather than to its absolute capacity. You perceive a lack of air when there is a reduction in your aerobic capacity from your own baseline. For example, an athlete who donates a pint of blood may still have twice the aerobic capacity of an untrained couch potato. This athlete, whose aerobic capacity has been reduced by anemia, may feel dreadful with exertion and be acutely aware that there's "not enough air." The couch potato, whose aerobic capacity is much smaller, but unchanged, may feel perfectly well and have no perception of any shortness of breath.

CAUSES

Dyspnea is an aerobic system problem. The sensation of difficulty is perceived to be in the lungs. The lungs may or may not be the problem.

In addition to the lungs, medical problems may also be caused by the heart, by a hormonal problem such as thyroid disease, or by a metabolic factor affecting oxygen delivery to muscle. Dyspnea may also be related to environmental, non-medical problems.

Lung problems include obstruction of airflow due to asthma, bronchitis, or

Figure 4-13

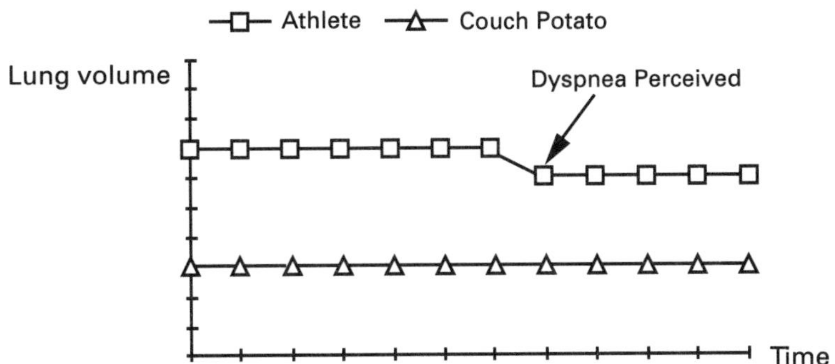

Dyspnea: Change in what is perceived, not absolute value.

emphysema. Blockage to the lung blood vessels, due to a clot, for example from a pulmonary embolus, commonly results in dyspnea. Diseases of the chest or respiratory muscles also cause dyspnea.

Heart disease in many forms is commonly associated with dyspnea.

An example of a metabolic factor causing dyspnea is anemia. The lack of oxygen carrying red blood cells results in an inadequate aerobic system. Shortness of breath with exertion may be the perceived symptom.

Environmental changes that cause dyspnea include riding at higher altitudes than usual and riding in polluted areas when one is unaccustomed to them.

TREATMENT

It is important to distinguish an abnormally uncomfortable awareness of breathing from the awareness of breathing all individuals experience with significant exertion. This is not a problem that lends itself to self-diagnosis. If you're bothered by your breathing, check with your doctor.

Exercise-Induced Bronchospasm

Many athletes complain of breathing problems during exercise. Some problems can occur under any circumstances; some are specific to exercise.

A FRAMEWORK OF LUNG PROBLEMS

The lungs, within the chest cavity, exchange oxygen from the air with carbon dioxide in the bloodstream.

You breathe in through your mouth and nose, and the air goes down your throat into the breathing tubes. From one big tube, which divides into two—one for each lung—the tubes get smaller and smaller. This allows an increase in the surface area available for interaction with the small blood vessels—the capillaries—of the lungs.

Greatly simplified, the common lung problems are these:

- Asthma—spasms of the air tubes
- Bronchitis—inflammation or infection of the air tubes
- Emphysema—destruction of the air tubes, usually from smoking
- Pneumonia—infection of the cells of the lung itself

Normal breathlessness that occurs when cycling hard usually has more to do with the heart, blood vessels, and muscle cells than it does with the lungs.

ASTHMA, BRONCHOSPASM, EXERCISE-INDUCED ASTHMA, EXERCISE-INDUCED BRONCHOSPASM (EIB)

Many people suffer from asthma, or spasm of the air passages. The classic definition of asthma used to be "reversible airway obstruction," implying that the spasm or obstruction of the air passages could be helped with medicines. The extent to which a lung problem could be reversed with medication reflected the degree of spasm. Modern thinking posits that in addition to pure spasm, some mucous-producing obstruction is involved. It's now known that some effects of asthma on lung function are irreversible in patients with long-standing disease.

Many individuals are aware that wheezing is the hallmark symptom of asthma. Cough, however, is the most common feature of this problem. Chest tightness is a frequent symptom.

Asthma shares the gene that predisposes a person to hay fever, allergic rhinitis (a nose condition), eczema (a skin condition), and migraine. When one or more of these medical problems runs in your family, you are more likely to have asthma, especially asthma made worse by allergies.

Many people have asthma as a child and "grow out of it." Others have mild symptoms related to their underlying tendency toward asthma—they may be aware that they wheeze only with a cold or the flu, or that their colds last longer than other people's.

Cold, exercise, dry air, and pollution are other factors that tend to bring on or worsen asthma. A cyclist often faces one or more of these exacerbants when riding. Many racers have problems with exercise-induced asthma, or exercise-induced bronchospasm (EIB). These terms are commonly used interchangeably. EIB affects perhaps as many as one-third of all racers and Olympic-endurance athletes.

HOW IS EIB DIAGNOSED?

Wheezing is the classical symptom. Chest tightness is often perceived. *Caution:* Heart disease may present similar symptoms. Sinusitis is sometimes misdiagnosed as a lung problem.

Everyone gets out of breath with significant exertion, so being out of breath is not in itself a reliable feature. With a big enough exertion, most people will cough after stopping, although those with exercise-induced bronchospasm will cough more frequently, longer, and after less exertion.

Those with EIB may find that cold weather makes them cough more readily, even without anaerobic efforts.

LUNG TESTS

A specific diagnosis can often be made with testing. This can be done with lung measuring equipment. These devices measure the force with which you can exhale, and then can show that exercise reduces this force. They can also demonstrate how medicines help restore or improve breathing.

Standard screening tests in many doctors' offices often don't uncover exercised-induced bronchospasm. Cyclists may have symptoms of EIB but also demonstrate normal or near-normal performance on screening lung function tests. Sometimes a test of lung function during or after exercise, or a trial of asthma medicine, may be necessary.

Here's an example. Figure 4-14 shows the results of forced exhalation spirometry, a lung test, of an elite woman bicycle racer. The little square boxes predict lung function, and her levels are above, or better than, those little squares.

The two most commonly used standard screening tests for lung function are the FEV_1, or forced expiratory volume in one second (how much air one can breath out in one second) and the FVC, or forced vital capacity (the total amount of air one can breath out). In Figure 4-14, the athlete's results are well above those predicted: 111% and 119% of normal. Most docs would say her test result is normal.

In my experience, the most important screening test is the third number listed in the figure. It's the FEF 25%–75%, or forced expiratory flow between 25% and 75% of the exhalation (the rate at which air is blown out in the middle part of the exhalation). You can't easily read it off the graph; it's computer generated. Hers is 85%. It's not bad, but not great.

Figure 4-15 shows what happened when I gave this cyclist an asthma medicine through a breathing machine and retested her lung function 30 minutes later. Her curve is even better, and we can see that her FEF 25%–75% rises from 85% of normal to 137% of normal—more than a 50% increase!

The good news: in her next race, an international stage race, this athlete easily placed in the top 10, feeling better than she had in months.

Figure 4-14

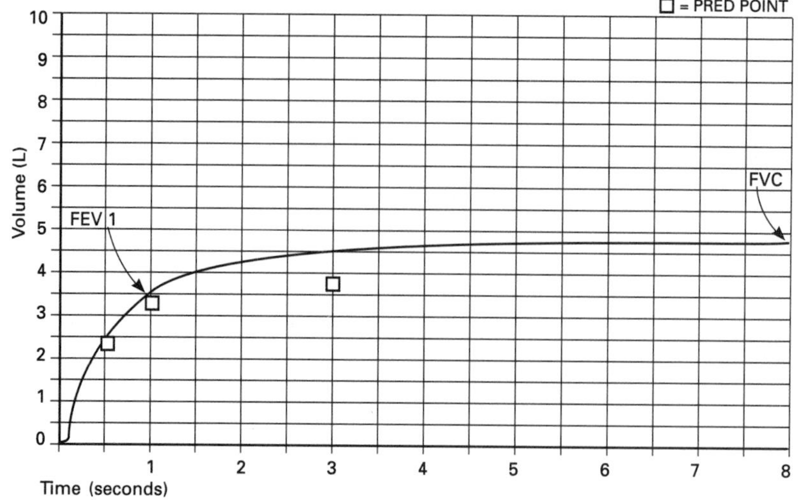

Measurement	Result	Predicted	% Predicted
FEV_1	3.74	3.37	111%
FVC	4.78	4.03	119%
FEF 25%–75%	3.25	3.83	85%

Spirometry before medication

TREATMENT FOR EXERCISE-INDUCED BRONCHOSPASM

- A gradual warmup helps prevent exercise-induced symptoms.
- Nose breathing, which helps increase the humidity of the air traveling to the lungs, may help.
- Avoid smog. See "Reducing Exposure to Pollution," below.
- Reduce exposure to common allergens and irritants. Common allergens include house mites found in house dust, flowers, certain weeds, trees, and cats. Common irritants include pollution, smoke, and home and workplace chemicals. Ammonia, for example, found in Windex and other cleaners, is a common home irritant.
- If you must be exposed to allergens and irritants, a face mask may help.
- Remember that other illnesses such as colds and the flu worsen asthma.
- Pre-exercise treatment with a variety of medications can help.
- Regular medication can reduce symptoms in those in whom simple pre-exercise medication is insufficient. Inhaled medicines are usually improperly or inadequately used. One-on-one instruction with a health-care professional is almost always required.

Figure 4-15

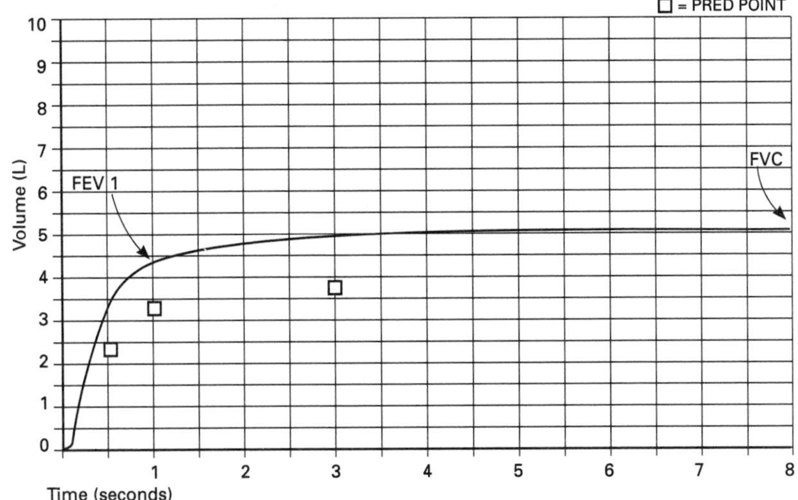

Measurement	Result	Predicted	% Predicted
FEV_1	4.38	3.37	130%
FVC	5.16	4.03	128%
FEF 25%–75%	5.26	3.83	137%

Spirometry after medication

MEDICINES USED FOR EIB

Various inhaled medications are used to help prevent or treat EIB.

The most common belong to a class of medicines known as *adrenergic agents*. All medicines in this group can cause anxiety, tremor, nervousness, or palpitations. These inhaler medicines are usually prescribed as such: two puffs, up to four times daily. If side effects are a problem, a single puff may be taken. The most frequently prescribed adrenergic medicine is albuterol (trade names Ventolin and Proventil).

Salmetrol (Serevent) is not marketed for EIB. It lasts longer than albuterol. Repeated overlapping doses have a potential for serious side effects. When it is used up to two puffs on days of competition, I have found it to be helpful and to produce fewer side effects. Over-the-counter epinephrine (Primatine) has more side effects than the adrenergic inhalers mentioned above. Use a prescription inhaler instead. *Cromolyns* (Intal, Tilade) are sometimes prescribed for EIB, but I have not found them as useful as the adrenergics.

Many patients often walk out of the physician's office with a prescription for an inhaled *steroid* (Beclovent, Vanceril, Azmacort, AeroBid). These medicines can be useful, but only if taken regularly, day after day. They are the drugs of choice for people who have persistent asthma (more than twice a week), but they do not work well with occasional use.

A common mistake is not receiving good instruction in the use of inhalers. In my experience, more than 75% of patients using inhalers do so incorrectly.

DRUG WARNING!

Some of the medicines used to treat EIB are banned by the United States Olympic Committee. Some are legal for use only if your physician registers you as a user.

Remember—there is a difference between medicines being dangerous and medicines being banned. If you need these medicines, registering their use is not bad—it only avoids the inference that you are using them for improved performance unrelated to a medical condition.

Although some athletes without EIB or asthma use these medicines for their perceived ergogenic benefit, it's doubtful that they are useful except to treat disease.

MONITORING EIB

Small hand-held peak airflow meters can be useful to help monitor asthma at rest and during rides. These devices cost about $25 and fit into a jersey pocket. They can be used at home to help monitor baseline lung function. They can be used on rides to give information about how exercise is affecting the lungs and how the lungs respond to medicine.

Reducing Exposure to Pollution

- Ride less-traveled roads. Stop-and-go traffic or busy roads are worse.
- Ride as far as possible to the right, out of the flow of traffic.
- Avoid peak traffic hours.
- Ride in the early morning rather than the late afternoon when pollution is worse.

Heart Symptoms

Heart disease may be a problem at any age, and it may strike even apparently fit young athletes.

One of the first things often recommended before you start up a vigorous exercise program is a medical checkup, especially if you are more than 40 years old. Just as many of us are quick to try our VCR or computer without instructions, many older riders begin their program and skip this step.

Whereas muscle or joint aches and pains are not likely to be catastrophic, ignoring a heart problem may be. You are much more likely to have heart disease if you have high blood pressure, are a smoker, have high cholesterol, or are diabetic. Men tend to get heart disease earlier than women, and those who are overweight or drink more than a couple of ounces of alcohol daily are also at risk.

Maybe you think it's heroic to start an exercise program without first having a medical checkup. If you have any of the warning signs of heart disease—such as chest pain or pressure, palpitations, or lightheadedness—and ignore them, you may become a dead hero. This is not a time for self-diagnosis. If the following problems occur and you are not sure what to do, see a doctor promptly if not emergently.

ANGINA

Angina is chest discomfort, pain, or pressure that results from insufficient blood supply to the heart muscle, usually caused by narrowing of the blood vessels that supply the heart—the coronary arteries. Although many lay persons presume that angina is perceived as pain, this is not always the case. Frequently angina is perceived as a weight, pressure, tightness, or smothering feeling on the chest.

Angina is usually centrally located on the chest, over a diffuse area. The sensation may radiate, or spread, toward the jaw, face, or arm, usually on the left side. Angina comes on suddenly, lasts at least several minutes, and gradually lessens. It is frequently brought on by exertion or emotion and relieved by rest.

Angina is a warning symptom of a heart attack. Do not ignore angina. See your physician.

PALPITATIONS

Everyone has an occasional "skipped" or irregular heartbeat. Persistent irregular beats, irregular beats associated with other heart symptoms, irregular beats associated with exercise, and irregular beats in those over 40 deserve evaluation by a physician.

UNEXPECTED HEART RATE CHANGES

Heart rate monitors allow athletes to observe their heart rates accurately. Everyone's heart rate monitor will occasionally register inaccurately. Battery, skin contact, and interference signals are some of the culprits behind registration errors. Sudden increases or decreases in heart rate without corresponding changes in exercise load, especially in older athletes or those with risk factors, may be a sign of heart disease.

LIGHTHEADEDNESS AND FAINTING

We all get lightheaded occasionally. Getting up quickly, dehydration, hot weather, alcohol, and emotion all increase the frequency of lightheadedness and fainting. Lightheadedness may also be related to decreased pumping action of the heart. This may be caused by an irregular heartbeat or by decreased muscle action of the heart.

REDUCTION IN WORKLOAD CAPACITY

Everyone experiences worsening performance at times. A decline in performance is often related to detraining or overtraining. Athletes who develop heart disease may also notice a decline in performance. In older athletes or those with risk factors, it may be a sign of worsening heart disease.

TREATMENT

Again, this is not a time for self-diagnosis or self-treatment. See a doctor promptly if not emergently.

Gastrointestinal Problems

What We're Talking About

Symptoms originating in the gastrointestinal (GI) tract that are related to exercise.

Of course, many gastrointestinal problems are not exercise-related—we're not talking about those here. Some gastrointestinal problems, such as diarrhea caused by infection with *Giardia* (which may be more common in Colorado mountain bikers), are also not discussed here. And although the problems listed here may be related to exercise, they may be caused by other problems. If symptoms are more than mild, or if bleeding is the symptom, seek medical attention.

More than one-third of participants in exhausting endurance events experience one or more of the following problems:

- GI shutdown: inability to take in fluids or solids
- Heartburn or other acid problems
- Diarrhea
- Cramps

- Nausea or vomiting
- Belching and gas
- Bleeding—hidden or apparent

GI Tract Changes with Exercise

During exercise, body functions change. It may take several hours after intense exercise for GI function to return to normal.

The following alterations occur:

- The normal emptying of the stomach is delayed.
- The stomach contents more easily back up into the esophagus—or food tube—than they normally do.
- Stomach acid secretion decreases.
- The normal movement of the GI tract—peristalsis—which propels food along, changes. Movement in the small intestine is slowed. Movement in the large intestine may increase.
- Blood flow to the GI tract decreases: more blood goes to the working muscles in the legs. Blood flow may be reduced up to 80%.
- Blood flow occasionally decreases so much that the lack of blood supply causes bleeding of the bowel wall or stomach.
- Nervous system activity changes.
- Substances in the circulation—for example, hormones and peptides—that affect the functioning of the GI tract, change.
- The absorption and secretion of substances in the lining of the GI tract change.

What Makes Things Worse

LEVEL OR INTENSITY OF EXERCISE

As exercise intensity increases, the physiologic changes described above increase. Whereas stomach emptying decreases by 80% or more with very high-intensity exercise, moderate exercise may decrease emptying by only 30%.

DEHYDRATION

When the exerciser is already dehydrated, there's less blood volume for the body to spare from exercising muscle. Dehydration causes a vicious circle: the more dehydrated you are, the more you need fluids, yet the harder it is for the gastrointestinal tract to accept them. The more dehydrated you are, the less well the stomach empties, and the less well the intestine absorbs the fluids you drink!

HEAT AND HUMIDITY

Another vicious cycle. Heat and humidity force the body to shunt blood to the skin to aid in cooling. Heat and humidity increase sweat rates and worsen dehydration. Both of these factors decrease the blood available to the gut. The need for fluids is increased, but the ability to handle them is worsened.

CONCENTRATED LIQUIDS OR SOLIDS

It is harder for your body to digest fluids or solids that are hyperosmolar (have a higher concentration than blood). The higher the concentration of fluids you drink, the harder it is for the body to process them. Before concentrated fluids can be absorbed, their concentration must be neutralized and must match the concentration of the blood. This means that the lining walls of the gut must secret fluids into the GI tract before the concentrated fluids you've consumed can be absorbed. Forcing the body to do this causes cramps, tightening of the gut, and diarrhea in many people. The energy bars and gels currently popular, when consumed without plenty of fluids, commonly cause these problems.

FRUCTOSE

Although fructose, or fruit sugar, has some important performance-enhancing properties, many find that fruit juices or sodas containing it are more difficult to tolerate than sports drinks containing glucose (table sugar).

FIBER, FAT, AND PROTEIN

All can contribute to gastrointestinal distress in susceptible individuals. In comparison with digestible carbohydrates, they slow the functioning of the gut and can cause digestive disorders.

CAFFEINE AND ALCOHOL

Caffeine and alcohol products cause many GI symptoms even in people who aren't exercising. They can certainly worsen symptoms in people who are.

ANXIETY

Just as caffeine and alcohol can cause many GI symptoms even in people who aren't exercising, we all know how anxiety or stress can tie our stomachs up in knots. Some riders become so nervous before important rides or races that they can't eat without distress for more than a day before the event.

What to Do—What Helps

PACE YOURSELF

Since increased exercise intensity worsens the functioning of the gut, it's prudent to pace yourself and not go out too hard. Consider a century ride. You could ride the first hour at 85% of your maximum heart rate, but your gut function would decrease substantially. Since you'll probably need to drink and eat to get even to the halfway point, it makes sense to ride closer to 75% of your max the first few hours, so that you'll be able to drink and/or eat.

HYDRATE

Remember, dehydration causes a vicious cycle. Keeping hydrated makes it easier to stay hydrated. If you start out well hydrated and then keep hydrated, it will be easier to sustain hydration.

DRINK TASTY COOL LIQUIDS

The stomach empties much faster with cool liquids than it does with warm liquids or those at air temperature. Some sugar and electrolytes in the solution improve its taste.

It's easy to prove this to yourself. After a long, hot ride, look at a warm jug of water. Then consider a big refrigerated bottle of Gatorade. Which looks more appealing? Try the water first. It won't take long before you've had enough. Next try the Gatorade. You can probably finish the whole bottle easily.

AVOID CONCENTRATED SOLUTIONS

A 5% glucose solution can empty five times faster from the stomach than a 40% solution and thus benefit the body more quickly.

AVOID CERTAIN FOOD AND DRINKS

There is a great deal of variability in what riders can successfully drink or eat. Some have success with certain drinks; others cramp up with the same ones. You've got to figure what works and what doesn't work for you. Full-strength fruit juices, some full-strength energy drinks, and fatty meals almost universally cause problems. Caffeine may help some riders perform, but it may cause GI symptoms in many others. Experiment on training rides, not during big events. In Europe, it's popularly believed that alcohol aids digestion; the reverse is often the case.

CONTROL YOUR ANXIETY

Perhaps easier said than done. Sometimes those new to racing just have to "get their feet wet" for their pre-race anxiety to disappear. Others may need to "give themselves a good talking to" and "get a grip" on things. Some athletes benefit from a sports psychologist who can help them constructively channel their anxiety.

TRAIN

Your gut probably doesn't get used to intense exercise, but training improves the ability of the gut to function at a given workload. With training, a smaller percentage of the exerciser's maximal oxygen uptake is required at any given workload, so that more is available for the GI tract.

Hemorrhoids

WHAT WE'RE TALKING ABOUT

Painful or itchy varicose veins at the end of the gastrointestinal tract, the anus. They may also bleed. They may be internal or external. The painful ones are usually caused by a blood clot in an external hemorrhoid.

CAUSES

Prolonged sitting, constipation, and pregnancy are associated with hemorrhoids. It's uncertain whether cycling causes hemorrhoids, but sitting in a saddle can certainly make them noticeable and uncomfortable.

TREATMENT

Most painful external hemorrhoids get better on their own. Hot (not burning) tub soaks may help. Creams may help the itch but are useless for pain. If you can't sit down, a relatively simple surgical procedure removes the clot and eases pain.

Cycling and Urination

What We're Talking About

Many cyclists notice that they seem to have patterns of urination related to their cycling. For example, it's common to hear riders say that they urinate more often when they've missed training for a few days or when they are overtrained. Or, riders say that once they start riding hard they never have to urinate again on that ride.

What's going on? What's the physiologic basis for these observations?

The Role of the Kidney

The kidney has two principal jobs: (1) to eliminate metabolic end-products, or waste, and (2) to regulate the volume and concentration of body fluids.

The kidneys eliminate metabolic end products such as urea, creatinine, urates, phosphates, nitrates, and sulfates. They regulate the concentration of sodium, chloride, bicarbonate, potassium, magnesium, and calcium as well as some metabolic end-products. The kidneys also regulate water to keep the body properly hydrated. They concentrate urine when the body is dehydrated and dilute urine when the body is overhydrated.

Cast of Characters—Kidney Function

The actual blood volume itself, metabolic waste products and blood chemicals, the nervous system, and various hormones all influence urine production.

BLOOD VOLUME

The higher the blood volume, the more the blood that flows to the kidneys. The more blood that flows to the kidneys, the more blood is filtered by the kidneys, and the more urine is formed.

METABOLIC WASTE PRODUCTS

The more metabolic waste products, the higher the solute load (the amount of chemical particles filtering through the kidney) and the more the kidney filters and eliminates. The more metabolic waste products, the more the kidneys need water to excrete them. For example, the reason that people with uncontrolled diabetes have increased urine volume is that high blood sugar levels perfusing the kidneys carry along water to eliminate the sugar.

THE NERVOUS SYSTEM

The sympathetic nervous system helps control the small blood vessels through a system of check valves located just before and just after the filtering mechanism of the kidney.

HORMONES

Hormones that affect kidney function include

- Aldosterone, produced by the adrenal glands, which increases during exercise and decreases the kidney's excretion of sodium
- Adrenaline and noradrenaline (also called epinephrine and norepinephrine), produced by the adrenal glands and sympathetic nerve endings, which increase during exercise and initially stimulate and then decrease urine production, increase heart output, increase circulating fatty acids, promote the breakdown of glycogen, and raise blood glucose
- Renin, produced by the kidneys, which stimulates the production of angiotensins, which in turn stimulate the production of aldosterone

- Vasopressin (also called anti-diuretic hormone, or ADH), produced by the posterior pituitary gland, which increases with exercise and slows urine production.

Cyclists' Blood Volume

With training, the amount of fluid in the blood vessels increases. With training, the numbers of red blood cells (RBCs) also increase, but to a lesser extent. Therefore, the percentage of RBCs may decrease.

Blood Volume During Exercise

A cyclist's blood volume during exercise decreases in proportion to the intensity of the exercise. Although the mechanisms are incompletely understood, a contributing factor is that compression of venous blood vessels in working muscles squeezes out fluid.

Urine Production During Exercise

With low-intensity exercise, blood flow to the kidneys increases. Since the blood flow increases, more urine is formed. With high-intensity exercise, blood flow is shunted to working muscles, and blood flow to the kidneys decreases. Less urine is made.

Role of Drugs

Many drugs affect urine production. Of course, prescription diuretics are used specifically to increase urine production. Over-the-counter substances also act as drugs. Caffeine and alcohol increase urine production.

Urination Frequency

Not urinating enough is a sign of dehydration, a common problem in athletes. Increased urinary frequency ("peeing often") can be due to either producing a large volume of urine, or urinating frequently with a small volume ("got to go, but a waste of time!").

Large-volume urination (having to go, having a lot to go each time), unrelated to cycling, is common in diabetes. It also occurs in persons who use diuretics or who overhydrate—compulsive water and coffee drinkers.

Cycling-related small-volume urinary frequency is commonly due to urethral irritation (irritation of the urinary passage in the penis or the urinary opening near the vagina) resulting from bicycle seat friction or pressure.

Women commonly have small-volume urinary frequency unrelated to cycling when they experience a urinary tract infection.

How Can I Avoid Urethral Irritation?

Get the pressure off your urethra and the front of your pelvis. Lower the nose of your saddle. Use a padded seat or one with a different shape. Place more weight on the back of your pelvis. Reduce riding time bent over in the handlebar drops—use the tops or hoods. Raise or shorten the stem. Stand periodically.

Is Psychology Involved?

You bet. It's common to perceive the need to urinate at the starting line of a race even though you've just been to the porta-pot five minutes before.

Once you've decided you've got to urinate while riding, it's hard to get your mind away from your bladder, even though in other circumstances you could easily "hold it."

Why Do I Urinate More When I've Missed Training?

Your blood volume is highest after you've missed a few days of training. Riding again provides a stimulus to reduce blood volume—the kidneys eliminate the excess.

Why Do I Urinate More When I First Start Riding?

Blood flow to the kidneys increases with low-intensity exercise. As you start warming up your kidneys produce urine more rapidly, and you have to urinate.

Why Do I Urinate Less During a Race?

As you race you generally get dehydrated. With high-intensity exercise, blood flow to the kidneys decreases, and urine production slows to a bare trickle. Also, your mind is more focused on other things.

How Can I Avoid Urinating in Long Races?

PERFECT SITUATION

Ideally, you start a race well hydrated and drink plentifully throughout the race. You know how to urinate off the bike while riding.

But life isn't ideal. Many riders must stop to urinate—they can't urinate while riding. Some men don't have the skill to liberate the penis and relax to urinate in the peloton, and both men and women are often unwilling to urinate into their shorts.

USE KIDNEY PHYSIOLOGY TO YOUR ADVANTAGE

- Hydrate the day before, not immediately before, a race. This will plump up the fluid reserves in your cells. If you hyperhydrate immediately before a race, your kidneys will sense the increased volume of your blood vessels and attempt to equalize it by continuing to form more urine even as the race proceeds.
- Warm up for half an hour at low intensity before long road races. This stimulates blood flow to the kidneys.
- Urinate before the race.
- Once you have been racing for 15 to 30 minutes, kidney blood flow is reduced. Less urine will be formed. Now is the time to start drinking to replace lost fluids.

Why Do I Urinate More When I Am Overtrained?

A few factors may combine to cause this phenomenon:

- You may attempt partial recovery by resting more and riding less, and so have a higher blood volume.
- Since you are tired, you may consume more stimulants, such as caffeine, which make you urinate more.
- You exercise at a lower intensity when overtrained, so that kidney blood flow may be increased, rather than decreased as it usually is with higher-intensity work.
- Hormonal and sympathetic nervous system stimulation of the kidney may be less functional, therefore, kidney blood flow may not be as reduced with exercise.
- You may drink more, either in the belief that you need fluids, because you ride less and have more time to drink, or because riding at a lower intensity allows you to do so. The more you drink, the more you urinate!

Diabetes

What We're Talking About

Diabetes is an endocrine (hormonal) problem in which either a lack of insulin or a lack of responsiveness to insulin results in several metabolic problems. Insulin is produced in the pancreas.

Most adults with diabetes are overweight. Weight reduction with diet modification and exercise will control or eliminate the signs and symptoms of diabetes in most of these individuals. Diabetics may take medicine by mouth to increase the body's responsiveness to the insulin it already produces, or may take insulin by injection to replace what is not made. Those who must take insulin in order to prevent relatively immediate, serious complications are classified as having insulin-dependent diabetes. Much of the discussion below concerns insulin-dependent diabetes. This information is not a substitute for individualized, professional, diabetic care.

What Insulin Does

Carbohydrates are digested and converted to simple sugars in the gastrointestinal tract. Simple sugars are then absorbed into the bloodstream. The actions of insulin result in the storage of blood sugar (glucose) in tissues. Insulin allows bloodstream sugar to be stored in the liver, muscle, and other areas as glycogen, or to be transported to adipose tissue and stored as fat.

The immediate problem for diabetics is high glucose levels in the blood. Without insulin, glucose stays in the bloodstream, and glycogen in muscle, liver, and other tissues is not made. Fat is overused as a source of energy, and ketones, acidic by-products of fat metabolism, accumulate in the blood.

Glucagon and Epinephrine

Balancing the role of insulin in lowering blood sugar, two other hormones—glucagon and epinephrine—raise blood sugar levels. Glucagon is also produced in the pancreas, and most insulin-dependent diabetics have a problem regulating this hormone.

Epinephrine (also called adrenaline) is produced by the adrenal glands. Insulin-dependent diabetics do produce this hormone, but epinephrine alone is often not sufficient to prevent low blood sugar.

Exercise Problems for Diabetics

Diabetics face several problems when they exercise. Exercise can result in blood sugar levels that are too low or too high.

Exercising muscles use glucose for energy. The demand for glucose during exercise in nondiabetics is met, in part, by decreased levels of insulin, which promotes liver glucose production and glucose release into the bloodstream for use by working muscles. Since exercise lowers blood sugar levels, insulin-dependent athletes who do not take this into account, by reducing the amount of injected insulin, risk low blood sugar, or hypoglycemia, the symptoms of which include sweating, nervousness, dizziness, tremor, hunger, weakness, palpitations, and headaches.

If exercise is begun with already high blood sugar (and low insulin) levels, exercise may worsen hyperglycemia (high blood sugar). Glucagon levels rise and increase liver glucose production. The already low insulin levels result in less glucose absorption and more fat-energy use by working muscles. Since high-intensity exercise is dependent upon glucose metabolism, performance will be impaired.

Since storage carbohydrate or glycogen is crucial for high-level performance, and since the making of glycogen is impaired in diabetes, high-level performance may be compromised even when blood sugar levels are optimum during exercise.

The kidneys help to normalize blood sugar levels by flushing out excess sugar. Their increased action in imperfectly controlled diabetes makes dehydration more likely.

Temperature regulation in diabetes is often impaired. Exercise in hot and humid conditions imposes additional demands and risks.

Benefits of Exercise for Insulin-Dependent Diabetics

- Improved control of blood sugar, including increased sensitivity of muscles to insulin, which may last for several days
- Reduced cardiovascular risks
- Weight loss
- Psychological benefits—stress reduction and a sense of well-being

Risks of Exercise for Insulin-Dependent Diabetics

- More difficult control, resulting in low and high blood sugars
- Delayed healing of orthopedic or foot injury
- Acceleration of degenerative joint disease
- Risk of worsening of high blood pressure
- Possible increased microvascular (including kidney and eye) complications

Types of Insulin and Usual Patterns of Use

The three most common types of insulin used are NPH (intermediate-acting), regular (short-acting), and lispro (rapid-acting). The key to understanding insulin use is understanding the pharmokinetics, or time-actions, of these products.

Table 4-2 **Pharmokinetic Characteristics of Three Common Types of Insulin**

	NPH	Regular	Lispro
Action	Intermediate	Short	Rapid
Onset	1 to 2 hours	15 to 45 minutes	0 to 15 minutes
Peak action	4 to 12 hours	2 to 5 hours	30 to 90 minutes
Duration of action	18 to 24 hours	6 to 8 hours	<5 hours

Many diabetics take a combination dose of NPH and regular or lispro insulin in the morning and at night. Typically, about 70% of the total daily dose is taken in the morning, and about 70% of each dose is NPH. A typical insulin-dependent diabetic might take 25/10 (25 units of NPH and 10 of regular or lispro) in the morning and 10/5 in the evening. Other diabetics take multiple daily injections before each meal and snack, or use an insulin pump, which supplies a continuous baseline amount of insulin as well as boluses (large one-time doses) before meals.

Energy Equivalents

A key to understanding control of diabetes is to think in terms of energy equivalents—the energy equivalent of food, exercise, and insulin. The information in these next few paragraphs is meant to be conceptual. Individual responses to insulin and exercise are quite variable. The only way athletes can really know by how much to adjust the insulin dose with exercise is by observing their own responses—through frequent measurement of blood glucose—to exercise, caloric intake, and insulin dose.

A typical, moderately active, cycling adult male insulin-dependent diabetic, weighing 70 kilograms, or 154 pounds, needs about 45 units of insulin daily.

These 45 units help manage a daily caloric intake of about 3,000 calories. Let us assume that this diabetic's diet is 60% carbohydrate—about 1,800 calories come from carbohydrates. One might then consider that each unit of insulin is equivalent to controlling 40 (1,800 divided by 45) carbohydrate calories of intake or that 1 unit of insulin is needed per 10 grams (40 calories) of carbohydrate.

Exercise has a caloric cost. At the high end of energy production, an elite-level professional male cyclist might continuously produce 400 watts of energy during a one-hour time trial. Since roughly 3 calories are needed for each watt-hour of energy production, this is equivalent to about 1,200 calories. Most of the calories used at this high level of exertion are carbohydrate calories.

A race-club rider might produce half as much energy per hour during a typical ride, or use about 600 calories each hour. If the club ride lasts for two hours, that's 1,200 calories. A hard 50-minute workout on a stationary trainer would also use about 600 calories per hour. A typical entry-level Category 4 or 5 road race or crit might use the same amount of energy. At this level, two-thirds of calories might be carbohydrate, one-third fat. Moderately easy riding might use half again as many calories, or 300 calories an hour. At this level, perhaps 40% of calories are supplied by carbohydrates and 60% by fat.

The use of 600 calories per hour represents about 400 carbohydrate calories, or about 10 (400/40) units of insulin. A rider planning to ride one hour at this level might therefore need about 10 fewer units of insulin during this hour ride.

At first consideration, one might think that the diabetic rider might also compensate by keeping the insulin dose the same and by consuming an additional 400 carbohydrate or 600 total calories per hour. The problem is that even under non-diabetic conditions, metabolism cannot work this fast to use ingested carbohydrate and/or fat. Working muscles can use only 200 to 250 calories per hour of ingested carbohydrate, or roughly half this amount.

The solution is straightforward. Insulin-dependent diabetics must reduce the dose of insulin that will be acting during their workouts. Diabetics (as well as non-diabetics) should consume about 250 calories per hour to help fuel their muscles directly.

Exercise Guidelines for Insulin-Dependent Diabetics

- Avoid beginning exercise with blood sugar levels below 70 mg/dL.
- Avoid beginning exercise with blood sugar levels above 300 mg/dL if ketones are present.
- Avoid dehydration. Drink before, during, and after exercise.
- Ingest 125 calories (about 30 grams) of carbohydrate for every 30 minutes of intense exercise.
- Have a recovery snack of carbohydrate after exercise.
- Decrease insulin dose by omitting regular or lispro insulin dose before exercise, decreasing your dose of intermediate-acting insulin the day of exercise, or, if using an infusion pump, eliminating the mealtime bolus preceding and following exercise.
- Be especially cautious about exercising at the peak of insulin action if no adjustment in insulin dose has been made.
- Avoid thigh injections of insulin for at least two hours before exercise.

Moderately Hard One-Hour Rides

After-breakfast morning or commute rides can be managed relatively easily if you omit the morning insulin dose of regular or lispro insulin and eat a little extra before, during, and after the ride.

Afternoon rides must be managed by reducing the morning NPH insulin dose. According to the energy-equivalent concept described above, a hard one-hour mid-afternoon ride may mean that only one-half of a typical 25-unit NPH dose should be taken.

Prolonged Rides

The absolute amount of stored liver glycogen cannot meet glucose demands for prolonged high-level performance, even in non-diabetics; fat metabolism becomes a factor. Just as non–insulin-dependent diabetics need to consume calories before, during, and after rides, so insulin-dependent diabetics need to try and optimize carbohydrate use for prolonged rides, not only to manage their diabetes but to increase performance.

Men's Health

Some bicycling problems are specific to men. Here are some issues of concern and suggestions for men's health.

Shaving Your Legs

You've decided to take the plunge and mow your legs.

WHY?

It's peer pressure. It's what racers do. Some say the aerodynamics are a little better, some say you can place dressings and bandages more easily in case of a fall, and some say massage is easier. Maybe. These benefits are marginal.

In the end, it really is a matter of peer pressure. After all, if no one else shaved their legs, you probably would feel pretty stupid doing it, wouldn't you? In fact, even with most racers shaving their legs, you may still feel self-conscious at company picnics or on the beach.

BLADES

If you are a shaving virgin, you need time—probably at least an hour. Most people use disposable blades and razors. Cheaper blades, such as those sold by BIC, cause more nicking. The best results come from double blades with a film of Teflon at one edge, such as Gillette Sensor blades.

In a shallow bath with warm water and soap, go to it. The first time will be slow. You'll have to rinse your blade frequently in order to shave. After that, successive shaves each week are much easier. Many riders find their weekly tub shave very relaxing.

ELECTRIC SHAVERS

Electric shavers have some advantages. Although electrics don't shave quite as closely, you don't need a bathtub or shower in order to shave. You can trim your growth every few days, or more often, without much fuss. You can save time by shaving while traveling, watching TV, or waiting for important faxes.

Electric shavers work by cutting your hair after the short stubs have penetrated the foil that covers the blades. If you let your hair grow too long, it's hard to use an electric efficiently. Most electrics have a trimmer originally designed for sideburns. Some of the Braun models have an adjustable height trimmer. Put up halfway, horizontal to the foil, it makes mowing your legs a snap. Even the initial deforestation can be accomplished in ten minutes.

HOW FAR?

Personal preference governs this decision. Obviously, you'd do well to shave at least an inch or two above your bicycle shorts line, or you'll look very strange. Shave higher if you wear street shorts that show more leg. If you swim in a Speedo, you've got to go all the way or you'll look very funny.

PROBLEM NICKS

Nicks are common with the disposables. Experiment with different blades.

MASSAGE PROBLEMS

Shaving your legs is supposed to facilitate massage. That may be true if you use oils or creams, as professional masseurs do. However, informal massage without oils or creams may actually be more difficult. Massage is ideally performed toward the heart. That's counter to the way hair is oriented on the legs, however, and unless the legs have been recently mowed, such massage can be irritating.

IRRITATED RED SPOTS

Folliculitis? Those little irritated red spots, especially near the crotch. Don't shave so high. Always shave in the direction of hair growth. Avoid Jacuzzis and tubs with jets that force surface bacteria into the skin. Diet, to lose weight, so that your legs don't rub together.

Penile Numbness

WHAT WE'RE TALKING ABOUT

Lots of men find that the penis feels numb or has a pins-and-needles sensation during or after riding. The penis may feel "asleep," swollen, or "not there." Usually just the shaft of the penis is the problem, but sometimes the numbness may extend to the scrotum and the base of the genitals. The problem is worse for longer rides, and worse after time trialing or riding for prolonged periods bent over in the drops or aero bars.

CAUSES

The cause is pressure on the pudendal nerve. The nerve gets compressed between the bicycle seat and the symphysis pubis of the pelvic bone. Debate exists whether the nerve itself is being compressed, or the small blood vessels that feed the nerve. Regardless, the effect is a disturbance in the functioning of the nerve and the tissues it supplies.

TREATMENT

The best treatment is prevention. The usual cause is riding bent over for too long. Take rests from this position. Stretch, and get the pressure off your genitals every five minutes by standing on the bike or otherwise changing your position.

Use a seat position that points the nose of the saddle down a little bit more, or lower the height of the seat. A padded or different saddle may be helpful—perhaps a differently shaped saddle with a different width. Padded bicycling shorts may help.

LONG-TERM COMPLICATIONS

Occasional nerve disturbance in this area usually resolves rapidly when pressure is relieved. Most riders regain normal sensation within minutes. Sometimes as much as twenty-four hours is required for the nerve to return to apparently normal function. Rarely more than a day is required. The longer it takes for the nerve to return to normal, the more damage is being done. Some small but real risk does exist for permanent damage unless you correct the problem.

This problem has nothing to do with the ability of your body to produce testosterone, the male hormone. It has nothing to do with your ability to produce sperm. But a numb penis is sometimes an "unfeeling" penis. Some men may have a problem with obtaining an erection, whereas others who achieve orgasm rapidly may find sexual relations improved because the reduced sensation helps them last longer.

Regardless, a numb penis should be avoided as much as possible because of the possibility of permanent nerve damage.

Penile Erection—Priapism

WHAT WE'RE TALKING ABOUT

Erection of the penis not related to sexual arousal.

CAUSE

The cause is the same as penile numbness, described above: pressure on the pudendal nerve.

TREATMENT

The treatment is the same as for penile numbness, described above: get the pressure off the pudendal nerve.

Impotence

WHAT WE'RE TALKING ABOUT

Impotence is the inability to obtain a satisfactory erection for sexual intercourse. It is not the same thing as infertility, which for a man means not having enough high-quality sperm. Bicycling is unlikely to cause permanent impotence. However, it is not unusual for riders to have occasional difficulties in sexual relations because of riding.

CAUSES

The ability to achieve a satisfactory erection for sexual intercourse depends upon several systems. The blood supply and the nerve supply to the genitals must be intact. The "most important sexual organ"—the brain—must also be in gear.

Sexual relations and achieving orgasm are similar to an interval on a bicycle. You need extra energy to achieve an erection and orgasm. If you are "totally wasted" after a very hard or long ride, you may not have the energy to engage in sexual activities. The inability to maintain a satisfactory erection often involves a combination of these factors.

Libido, or the interest in sexual relations, is dependent upon many factors, including testosterone. Studies have shown that during racing season, athletes have decreased levels of testosterone, in part related to exertion, and in part related to weight loss and a low percentage of body fat. These factors, combined with the general exhaustion of training and racing, often result in decreased sexual activity.

Bicycle seat pressure can reduce nerve conduction to the penis. Decreased sensation in the penis can contribute to reduced sexual performance. This problem is usually a temporary one, although accident and injury can cause prolonged problems. There are a few reports of prolonged nerve damage from prolonged pressure.

TREATMENT

Avoid excessive compression of the genitals and nerve injury through proper bicycle position. Consider modifying your training or sexual schedule if you find that the energy required to perform both activities is too much within a given period of time. Understand the physiologic effects of significant training on your overall energy level and libido.

Infertility—Sperm Abnormality

The many causes of infertility in men are not discussed here. It is not common for cycling to be the problem.

Sperm, which are made in the testicles and travel through the epididymis and vas deferens of the scrotum, need the proper temperature to function optimally. Normally, the testicles are pulled closer to the heat of the abdomen in cold conditions and "hang loose" in hot conditions. Exercise and tight cycling shorts may result in scrotal overheating and poor sperm function. This is an occasional cause of infertility and is almost always correctable. High-volume high-intensity athletes have lowered testosterone production. This can lead to reduced sex drive and reduced frequency of intercourse.

Bloody Semen

Bloody semen without significant blood in the urine is usually related to the breakage of a small blood vessel, often within the prostate. It is rarely related to any significant medical problem. Although some physicians tell their patients not to worry about this problem and don't even examine them for it, if you are over 40 or if the problem persists for more than a week, it is reasonable to check with your physician.

Bloody Urine

Although this problem can occur in athletes for reasons unrelated to any medical condition, it is always wise to consult a physician. It has been reported that pressure on the urethra or bladder tube can cause bloody urine, but it is more likely that it is unrelated to cycling and warrants the same medical evaluation as bloody urine in non-cyclists.

Urinating While Riding

In long road races you will almost always see some guys relieving themselves while riding the bicycle. How do they do it? You may have tried it once or twice but found it difficult.

ON-THE-BIKE POTTY TRAINING

- Choose a quiet road where you won't offend pedestrians or others.
- Choose a flat or slightly downhill section.
- Liberate your penis—either above the top or down the leg of your shorts.
- Don't have your penis confined and partially bent or compressed by your shorts.
- Visualize yourself at a urinal, not on your bike.
- Relax.
- See yourself urinating freely in the urinal.
- Practice alone.
- Practice with a trusted friend.
- Maybe soon you'll be ready for the peloton!

Condom catheters—condoms with a tube at the end—can be rolled up on the penis and the tube left to dangle outside of a pant leg, allowing urination for those who find the above method too difficult. This can be a little messy.

Urinating Difficulties

Cycling-related pressure leading to inflammation of the urethra or bladder tube may cause frequent urination, dribbling, decreased urinary stream force, nighttime urination, or burning upon urination. Additionally, an infection can be a complication of this irritation. Pressure on the pudendal nerve, which can cause penile numbness, can decrease sensation during urination.

Riders over 40 may have difficulties related to the prostate. Hesitancy before urinating and dribbling after urinating are also common problems with the prostate and are, for many men, a "normal" part of aging. Since other medical conditions may also cause these problems, it's wise to check with your physician if you experience them. It is controversial whether cycling aggravates the prostate.

Pressure can be relieved by varying position, by using padded saddles, by using wider tires with lower air pressure, by using suspension, or by using less stiff bicycles or recumbents.

Prostatitis

Prostatitis is an inflammation of the prostate gland. The prostate is a walnut-sized organ between the rectum and the urethra, or bladder tube.

True medical prostatitis is often caused by a microorganism that brings about an infection and is treated with antibiotics. Since it is difficult for antibiotics to enter the prostate gland, treatment with antibiotics usually is given for many weeks to prevent recurrence. An ache in the prostate area is not necessarily related to infection at all. Perhaps a chronic swelling of the prostate is responsible. Bacterial debris may cause a chronic immunologic reaction. Or perhaps, as in many headaches and stomachaches, there is no disease to be found but the problem is related to stress or other unknown factors.

Although pressure on the prostate is said by some to result from bicycle riding and to cause or aggravate typical prostate symptoms, many physicians doubt this and find no scientific evidence to support the hypothesis. Most physicians doubt that infection of the prostate is related to cycling. Cancer of the prostate is not related to cycling.

Swollen Testicles

Swelling in the testicles is often due to inflammation of the epididymis, the collecting system for sperm at the back of the testicle, and not truly swelling of the testicle itself. Most often this problem is infectious and can be treated with antibiotics. Any swelling in the genitals should prompt consultation with a physician. Cancer of the testicle, although unlikely, can occur in younger as well as older men.

Vasectomy

Cycling can normally be resumed one week following vasectomy.

Women's Health

Some bicycling problems are specific to women. Here are some issues of concern and suggestions for women's health.

Nipple Friction and Pain

Riding sometimes results in irritation of the nipples. Clothing chafes at the skin and causes irritation. Once irritation occurs, repeated rubbing only worsens the problem. Wet clothes are especially irritating.

A support bra may help. Wearing a lightweight undershirt under your jersey reduces skin rubbing and relieves irritation. Sometimes a Band-Aid covering helps a particularly irritated nipple. An emollient, such as Vaseline, may protect the skin and reduce irritation. Wear layers, dress appropriately to the weather, and change out of wet clothes as soon as possible.

Bicycle Seat Discomfort

Most of us are aware that the shape of a woman's pelvis is different from that of a man's. In fact, there are three or four common shapes to the pelvises of women, and some women do have an android shape similar to that of men. For this reason, the shape of a saddle that will provide the most comfort is an individual affair. Whereas most men will find the same kinds of saddles comfortable, this is not the case for women. You will probably need to try saddles of different shapes to determine the type that best matches your anatomy.

Seats: padding or no padding, gel-filled or not? The answers to these questions depend upon your riding style and the type of riding you do. Some saddles, such as the Terry, have a wide acceptance with many women. Some thin seat covers, such the one made by Pearl Izumi, allow an extra layer between you and the saddle to absorb rubbing, preventing your own anatomy from being chafed.

Sometimes problems of seat comfort are related to the general fit of a bicycle. Most bicycles are designed for men. Most bikes are sized with too long a top tube. This too-stretched-out position can make the seat uncomfortable near the pubic bone.

Seat position traditionally has been with the nose of the saddle pointed slightly up or level. Some women need the nose pointed just slightly down in order to be comfortable and avoid irritation of the urethra—the tube that carries urine from the bladder. The time-trialing position is the worst for most women. Improved flexibility may allow you to rotate your pelvis as you ride, reducing pressure on your pubic area while at the same time allowing you to bend over and achieve a more aerodynamic position.

A numbing cream may occasionally be used in this area.

Sex Before or After Bicycling

For many women, riding places pressure on the vaginal and pubic areas. This pressure may result in local inflammation or irritation, including swelling and chafing. Since sexual activity often also places pressure on these areas and may cause similar soreness due to inflammation, some women have discomfort when they ride after sexual activity, and some women have difficulty with sexual activity soon after riding.

Placing more pressure on your buttocks and away from the pubic area may be helpful. If you anticipate sexual activity after a ride, you may wish to spend more time riding on the tops than in the drops. Make sure that your bike fit is correct, that you are not too stretched out, and that the nose of your saddle isn't too high, thereby irritating your pubic area. A different saddle may help.

Vulvar Swelling

Women who spend a lot of time on the saddle occasionally develop swelling of the external genital area, the vulva, usually on one side. Pain is not usually a problem. The cause of the condition is not precisely known.

Since this is not considered dangerous or worrisome, the solution—reducing saddle time—has not usually been of much interest to most of the patients I have seen.

Yeast Infections

Vaginal yeast infections are often caused by an overgrowth of *Candida* yeast, which is normally found in small quantities in the vagina. Factors that contribute to this overgrowth include the use of oral antibiotics and increased warmth and moisture.

Reduce the warmth and moisture in this area. Read the paragraphs about warmth and moisture in the chapter "Crotchitis," beginning on page 185.

Regular douching is not healthy for the vagina, although an occasional vinegar douche is not harmful. Over-the-counter vaginal anti-yeast cream, for example, Gyne-Lotrimin, may be helpful.

Not all vaginal infections are caused by yeast. If you are not sure or if the problem does not clear up with self-treatment, see your doctor.

Uterine Cramps

Menstrual cramps are familiar to most women. Occasionally, uterine cramps occur with exertion and are not related to menstruation. Like menstrual cramps, exercise-induced uterine cramps may be helped with two to four tablets of Advil—that is, 400 to 800 mg of ibuprofen. This dose may be taken three or four times a day for several days each month. Other prescription non-steroidal anti-inflammatory drugs may also work. Read the chapter about NSAIDs, beginning on page 161.

The most common side effect of anti-inflammatory drugs is abdominal discomfort. If this becomes a problem for you, stop the medicine.

Pregnancy

There is no good scientific proof that riding while a woman is pregnant is either good or bad. Pregnancy does increase the physiologic demands on the body. It makes temperature regulation more difficult, and excessive heat may be harmful to the developing fetus. It reduces the amount of glycogen and energy you will have for cycling. As your abdomen becomes larger your center of gravity rises, and balance will be more difficult. Avoid situations that put you at risk for falling.

Assuming you have not had any problems with past pregnancies or your current one, you probably can ride normally for the first six months of your pregnancy as long as you limit your exertions to 80% of your maximum heart rate and avoid overheating. After six months of pregnancy, many women feel awkward on a bicycle and don't want to risk falling. Stationary bicycles are an alternative. It is probably wise to limit your prolonged exertions to 70% of your maximum heart rate.

Bladder Infections

Most women know the feeling of burning and frequent urination that comes from a bladder infection. Such infections are usually caused by *Escherichia coli,* a bacterium commonly found in stool. It is a short distance from the anus to the urethra—the bladder-emptying tube. The urethra in women is also very short, and once the urethra has been colonized by bacteria, a bladder infection develops easily. Wiping in the wrong direction, certain sexual practices, and bicycle riding may all allow these bacteria easier access to the urethra and the bladder.

AVOIDING BLADDER INFECTIONS

- Avoid dehydration. Drinking often results in frequent urination, which may help wash out bacteria, allowing the body to reduce the numbers of bacteria on its own. Concentrated urine stings and causes symptoms that may be mistaken for a bladder infection.

- When you have to urinate, don't procrastinate. Procrastination may allow the bladder to swell, reducing the amount of blood that nourishes it, making it more prone to infection.
- Urination after sexual activity and riding reduces bladder infections.
- Avoid pressure on the pubic area by using the correct seat position.
- An acid urine prevents bacterial growth. One way to keep the urine healthy and acidic is to take 1 gram of vitamin C (ascorbic acid) daily. Alternatively, approximately 1 gram of aspirin—three regular-strength tablets—will also help acidify the urine.

Pressure or chafing irritation of the end of the urethra due to seat position may cause the same symptoms without a true bacterial infection. This is similar to "honeymoon cystitis," which sometimes isn't an infection at all but rather an irritated urethra that hasn't adapted to sexual activity.

Alternatively, the irritation may weaken the surface of the urethra, allowing bacteria to grow, and resulting in an infection.

TREATMENT

Prescription antibiotics are very effective for bladder infections. Prompt cure of this problem can be expected in almost all patients.

Tampon Hints

Don't leave the string outside the vagina when you ride. It is often rubbed by the saddle, and the chafing frequently causes irritation. If your flow is so heavy that one tampon is insufficient, try using two tampons side by side at the same time. This can be much more comfortable than using a tampon with a pad.

Too Thin?

It was once said that you can't be too rich or too thin. Is this true? Not as far as weight is concerned. You *can* be too thin, and you can be a poorer rider or racer because of excessive leanness. There are other health consequences of too little fat, especially for women.

TOO THIN CAUSES PROBLEMS

There is no question that someone with a spare tire would do well to shed those love handles. Excessive fat is just extra poundage you have to lug up hills, accelerate to speed with jumps, and otherwise metabolically support.

Excessive leanness, on the other hand, probably hampers your immune system and lowers your resistance, making you more susceptible to colds, flu, and other infections. It may inhibit recovery and fosters greater fatigue. Especially in women, excessive leanness is associated with eating disorders, menstrual irregularities or the loss of menstruation, and osteoporosis.

THE "TOO-THIN" TRIAD

The female athlete "too-thin" triad consists of disordered eating, amenorrhea (loss of periods), and osteoporosis. Some studies have shown that over one-half of athletic women have components of this triad. Old bones in young athletes are a serious problem. More information is found in the next chapter, "Osteoporosis."

BODY FAT GOALS

A reasonably ideal body fat for a top-level female racer is 10% to 15%; for a top-level male racer it is 5% to 10%. Some women do get down to 6% to 8% and some men down to 3% to 4%. Such leanness isn't for everyone.

If you are always tired, cranky, or overstressed, consider letting your weight rise a few pounds and see if you feel better. Women thin enough to have lost their periods should consider supplementing their diets with extra calcium and hormone treatment—most easily available in the form of birth control pills—to help prevent osteoporosis.

Leanness can improve athletic performance, but that doesn't mean it's healthy.

Osteoporosis

WHAT WE'RE TALKING ABOUT

Osteoporosis—low bone density, or thinning of the bones—is a common health problem in women, especially after menopause, and an occasional problem in men. Weakened bones are more likely to break. Endurance and high-intensity cyclists often have irregular menstrual periods and altered hormonal status, which places them at risk for osteoporosis and future bone fractures.

Women often know their weight, blood pressure, cholesterol level, and percent body fat. They often don't know the status of their bone health.

RISK FACTORS

- Reduced cumulative estrogen exposure from any of the following: delayed onset of menstruation, early menopause, absent or irregular periods
- Family history of osteoporosis or a history of low bone density
- Nutritional deficiencies, including low intake of calcium and vitamin D; eating disorders; and low calorie intake
- High level of physical activity

- Thin, small body
- White or Asian race
- Stress or low-trauma fractures
- Medications, including thyroid hormone replacement, corticosteroids, and phenytoin
- Smoking
- High alcohol intake
- High caffeine intake
- Diseases, including intestinal malabsorbtion

DIAGNOSING OSTEOPOROSIS

A woman of any age who has prolonged estrogen deficiency (resulting in irregular or absent periods) or other risk factors should consider taking a bone density measurement for evaluation of her bone health. Bone density can be measured at various sites and by various technologies. If only one measurement is made, the site usually examined is the lumbar spine in women younger than 65 and the femoral neck in women 65 and older.

PREVENTION AND TREATMENT

- *Nutrition.* Calcium intake of 1,500 milligrams daily. Calcium can be obtained from the diet or from supplements. Dairy products, dried beans, sardines, and broccoli are high in calcium. Vitamin D helps calcium absorption.
- *Improved estrogen levels.* Before menopause, reduced exercise duration or intensity, increased caloric intake, or estrogen replacement with oral contraceptives may help. After menopause, estrogen replacement therapy (ERT) has been shown to prevent osteoporosis.
- *Weight-bearing exercise.* Weight lifting and walking are associated with improvement. Cycling is not weight-bearing. Long-distance cycling is associated with a worsening of osteoporosis.
- *Smoking cessation.*
- *Medical prescription therapy.* New therapies, in addition to estrogen, include bisphosphonates and calcitonin. Ask your doctor.

Estrogens, Birth Control Pills

Estrogens are female hormones that the body produces. The supraphysiologic amounts in birth control pills suppress ovulation. Replacement estrogens are frequently prescribed for postmenopausal women when their naturally occurring levels wane.

There are pluses and minuses in the use of estrogens. They may slightly decrease aerobic metabolism and promote fluid retention, and thereby adversely affect performance. When given to postmenopausal women without progesterone, estrogens slightly increase the risk of uterine cancer. This risk is minimized by using progesterone as well.

Estrogens significantly reduce osteoporosis and cardiovascular disease. They may reduce the risk of Alzheimer's disease. Birth control pills usually reduce menstrual bleeding and are associated with a reduced amount of anemia. They often help menstrual irregularities and cramps, allowing athletes to train more consistently and predictably.

Part Five

GENERAL HEALTH

The General-Health Exercise Prescription

The exercise prescription includes aerobic, resistance, and stretching components.

Aerobic exercise—such as bicycling, brisk walking, jogging, running, swimming, aerobics, or rowing—should be performed on most, if not all, days each week. Work out at least twenty minutes per session. Begin and end with a warmup and a cooldown. People who have previously been inactive should begin at a comfortable pace for twenty minutes, three times per week. Gradually increase time, frequency, and intensity.

Resistance exercise should be performed two to three times each week, using free weights or machines. Perform progressive resistance exercises with instruction and supervision until the techniques have been mastered.

Stretching exercises should be performed after each aerobic and resistance session to improve and maintain flexibility. Perform them under supervision until the techniques have been mastered.

Those who have any medical problems or symptoms (e.g., chest pain, shortness of breath, fainting, diabetes, asthma) should be medically evaluated before starting any exercise program. Prevention of obesity, osteoporosis, cardiovascular disease, and adult-onset diabetes is a sufficient incentive to keep most adults exercising—especially when the activities are enjoyable.

Exercise Addiction

What We're Talking About

Too much of a good thing. I'm an exercise advocate for those who enjoy exercising. But just like anything else, too much exercise can be a problem.

Signs and Symptoms of Exercise Addiction

- Recurrent overuse injuries
- Refusal to discontinue exercise even when pain or discomfort is associated with the exercise
- Neglecting family or work to spend time exercising
- Loss of enjoyment when exercising
- Excessive concern about body image, weight loss, eating disorders
- Resistance to cutting back; denying there is a problem
- Withdrawal symptoms including depression, anxiety, and guilt

Treatment

As with most addictions, the first step is often recognizing that there is a problem. Professional counseling may be helpful.

Fatigue — Why Am I Tired?

Riders may find themselves tired and wonder why. Your tiredness probably falls into one of these categories:

- Stress, emotional turmoil
- Inadequate sleep
- Too rapid weight loss
- Inadequate nutrition
- Medical problems, including depression
- Overtraining/burnout

Stress

Stress is one of the most common reasons why athletes and nonathletes alike are tired. Most people think of stress as bad events in their lives. Actually, stress is change.

Good changes and bad changes are stressful. Getting a new bicycle and figuring out all the components you want to put on it and being excited about it may be good, but your increased anxiety may cause you to lose sleep and get exhausted just in planning—never mind riding—your new bike! Marriages, separations, deaths in the family, job changes, new purchases, and accidents are some of the big stresses in our lives. Get too many of them in a year and most of us become tired, perhaps as a psychological way of avoiding these stressful situations.

Consider the important people and things in your life: family and friends, job, money, lover(s). Have these changed recently? If so, stress may contribute to your fatigue.

Inadequate Sleep

Sleep loss is an understandable cause of fatigue. Inadequate sleep is often related to the stresses already discussed. By going to sleep at a regular hour and arising at a regular hour, you set the pattern for good sleep habits. Quiet activity fifteen minutes before sleep—reading a book or listening to soft music—may also help you sleep better.

Too Rapid Weight Loss

Many athletes rightly try to lose weight to improve their performance. Weight loss of more than one to two pounds weekly, though, often results in fatigue and worsens performance.

Inadequate Nutrition

Your body needs calories, nutrients, and fluids to work properly. If you ride for more than a couple of hours and get tired, the problem may be simply that you need to eat and drink more! Chronic glycogen depletion is a common cause of fatigue. Read more about this in the chapter "Diet: Why High Carbohydrates?," beginning on page 9.

Medical Causes

If your fatigue lasts more than a month or two, a medical checkup may be wise. Some causes include anemia, diabetes, low thyroid, other organ disease of almost any kind, infectious diseases, and depression.

Depression is an extremely common medical illness characterized by fatigue and irritability. Although emotional lows or sadness may be present, many people with medical depression do not report these feelings. Interrupted sleep, change in sex drive, pain, lack of enjoyment, change in bowel habits, difficulty with concentration, and feelings of worthlessness also characterize depression. These symptoms often overlap with those of overtraining, which is discussed below. Depression is very effectively treated with medication—antidepressants.

Chronic fatigue syndrome is a poorly understood medical condition. No consistent physical findings, laboratory tests, causes, or treatments exist. As is the case with other medical problems that remain poorly defined, personal testimonial and anecdotal reports, often presented with considerable conviction, cloud the scientific evidence. At one time, Epstein-Barr virus was thought to be related to this problem. Current evidence dismisses this possibility. Some patients' symptoms may be improved by the simple addition of salt to the diet. It is clear that depression is often present.

Overtraining or Burnout

What We're Talking About

Fatigue, apathy, lethargy, or staleness in otherwise healthy athletes.

Think of overtraining as a physical situation, burnout as a psychological or emotional one. They are intertwined, since most psychological states have a physical, biochemical, metabolic, and/or neurohormonal basis. Overtraining is an imbalance between training and recovery, exercise and exercise capacity. The "training effect" is the body's response to workload stress. If stress is too great, the body cannot respond and adapt. Overtraining may result.

A note about terminology: *Overloading* is a building or anabolic adaptation to workload stress. *Overtraining* is breakdown or catabolic response. *Overuse* is musculoskeletal overtraining.

The trick in maximizing human performance is to perform the greatest volume of intense training without overtraining. Some say: "Put your finger near the fire to know that it is hot, but do not burn it!" Push, yes, but not too hard all the time. You need some easy days, some quiet friendly rides, maybe some bike touring. Ignore recovery training, and you may dig yourself a hole that not even a week or two off the bike can cure—then you may really lose fitness!

If you go from 100 to 200 miles in a couple of weeks, you may be mentally eager to ride more, but your body may say no. It is important to have a measured increase in workload to avoid fatigue. If you increase your mileage more than 10% per week, you should cut back on intensity, or you're likely to become tired.

You may be enthusiastic about getting stronger, and read a program on interval training. If you begin a serious program of interval training, even with a good base, it is difficult to maintain such a program without diversity and measurable results, or other positive feedback. If you do the same workouts day in, day out, even though they may be physiologically sound, it's easy to suffer burnout.

My rule of thumb is this: "When you look at the bike in the morning, are you raring to get on it or do you groan inside about the workout you have set for yourself?"

Overtraining symptoms include the following:

- Poor, non-restorative sleep
- Mood disturbances, including anxiety, irritability, loss of enjoyment, and sadness
- Poor performance with the same or increased training
- Vague or undefined physical complaints

Stress in Athletes

A combination of training and non-training stresses affect athletes.

Training stresses include

- Too much volume
- Too much intensity
- Too little recovery

Common situations that result in training stress include

- Excess competition
- Attempts to follow a training plan when injured or ill
- Inappropriate increased training in an attempt to make up for rest related to injury or illness
- Inappropriate increased training in an attempt to make up for poor competition performance

Non-training stresses include

- Excessive work, school, or family responsibilities
- Interpersonal conflict with co-workers, bosses, friends, or family
- Drug problems
- Housing problems
- Money problems
- Legal problems
- Illness or injury in self or others
- Insufficient sleep
- Poor diet

Short- and Long-Term Overtraining

Short-term overtraining may be related to local muscle factors, including depletion of glycogen or muscle injury. Long-term overtraining involves, in addition, neurohormonal factors in the nervous system, including the brain and the endocrine glands.

Short-term overtraining, also called overreaching or isolated peripheral overtraining, is characterized by the following:

- Development over a few days to two weeks
- Exercise fatigue
- Reduction in submaximal performance capacity
- Reduction in maximum performance capacity
- Short-term inability (desire and physical capacity) to compete
- Recovery achieved within days
- Favorable prognosis

Long-term overtraining, also called overtraining syndrome, staleness, or combination peripheral and central overtraining, is characterized by the following:

- Development over a few weeks to months
- Exercise and non-exercise fatigue
- Reduction of submaximal performance capacity
- Reduction of maximum performance capacity
- Mood disturbance
- Muscle soreness/stiffness
- Long-term inability (desire and physical capacity) to compete
- Recovery requiring weeks to months
- Uncertain prognosis

How Is Overtraining Diagnosed?

Clinical symptoms, athletic performance, and medical tests point the way to the diagnosis. No test is foolproof or perfect. For most symptoms and tests, other medical conditions give similar profiles.

In self-monitoring, the best-known markers to watch for are these:

- Morning weight down more than 3%
- Hours of sleep down more than 10%
- Resting heart rate increased more than 10%
- Mood changes including fatigue, loss of enthusiasm, and depression

Research suggests that with overtraining, relative to otherwise healthy adaptation, these things occur:

- Maximum heart rate decreases.
- Hormones change. Cortisol: resting and 8 A.M. blood levels of cortisol increase; post-exercise blood levels decrease. Catecholamines: levels decrease in urine at night by more than 50% and increase relatively more for the same intensity of exercise. Testosterone levels in blood decrease. Insulin responsiveness decreases.
- Blood chemistries change. Triglycerides, low-density lipoprotein lipids, and very-low-density lipoprotein lipids decrease. Maximum lactate and submaximum lactate decrease. Submaximum levels may (falsely) give the impression of improved performance. The ratio of blood lactate to perceived exertion decreases. Glutamine use decreases.
- Neurotransmitters change. Serotonin levels in the brain increase.
- Immunoglobins and the immune system changes. Immunoglobulin A (IgA) in saliva decreases.
- Muscle energy and water stores change in short-term overtraining syndrome. Glycogen is depleted, and intracellular stores of water are reduced.

Avoiding Overtraining

- Individualize training.
- Do not increase frequency, duration, or intensity too quickly.
- Allow for recovery. Plan and schedule rest days.
- Build up a good endurance base before undertaking interval work.
- Sleep at least eight hours a night.
- Consider afternoon naps, rest, or meditation.
- Review non-training stresses, and attempt to reduce or accommodate them.
- Avoid overcompensating for time missed from training.
- Avoid overcompensating for poor race performance.
- Adjust your goals.
- Eat a nutritionally sound high-carbohydrate diet to help prevent glycogen depletion.
- Hydrate.
- Monitor your morning pulse, weight loss, and sleep patterns for self-diagnosis of overtraining.

Medication: Depression and Overtraining

Symptoms, athletic performance, and medical tests are often the same or overlap considerably in overtraining and medical depression. Some believe that overtraining is a cause of medical depression. Medical depression also lessens the ability to train. Preliminary scientific investigation suggests that antidepressant medication may help athletes train harder, treat overtraining syndrome, and improve their performance.

Exercise and Immunity

The effects of aerobic exercise in general, and of bicycling in particular, on the immune system are uncertain. The study of the immune system is in its infancy. Preliminary information suggests that the short-term effect of exercise is a lowering, or worsening, of the immune system. Long-term regular exercise may help the immune system.

The strength of the immune system appears to decline with age. Some of this decline may be offset by a program of lifelong, regular aerobic exercise.

Anemia

Transport of oxygen, transport of carbon dioxide, and buffering of acids—these are vital functions that must operate optimally for an athlete to demonstrate peak performance. If you are anemic, this will be a problem.

What We're Talking About

Anemia is a deficiency of the red blood cells—usually a lack of cells. Occasionally, a problem with cell function makes the situation worse.

The main function of the red blood cell is to transport hemoglobin, the blood protein that carries oxygen from the lungs to the tissues. Red blood cells also contain the enzyme carbonic anhydrase, which speeds up the reaction between carbon dioxide and water. This reaction helps the blood transport carbon dioxide from the tissues to the lungs.

Hemoglobin is also an excellent acid-base buffer. Buffering is necessary to help neutralize exercise-produced lactic acid. Red blood cells are responsible for about 70% of the buffering power of the blood.

Anemia is usually determined by analyzing blood for the amount of hemoglobin or the percentage of red blood cells it contains.

Blood Tests in Anemia

1. *Hemoglobin (Hgb):* the quantity of hemoglobin in a sample of blood measured in grams per deciliter.
2. *Hematocrit (Hct):* the percentage of blood made up of red blood cells.
3. *Serum iron:* the amount of iron in the blood, measured in micrograms per milliliter.
4. *Ferritin:* a form of storage iron, measured in nanograms per milliliter.

Table 5-1 **Normal Values of Blood Tests**

	Male	Female
Hgb	13 – 18 g/dL	11.5 – 16.0 g/dL
Hct	39 – 54%	35 – 48%
Serum iron	40 – 170 μg/mL	40 – 170 μg/mL
Ferritin	20 – 450 ng/mL	10 – 350 ng/mL

How Red Blood Cells Are Made

Red blood cells are produced in the bone marrow. Not enough red blood cells means that not enough oxygen can be transported. Too many red blood cells increase the thickness of the blood and slows blood flow. The numbers of red blood cells that are produced are regulated by the amount of oxygen that reaches the tissues. Lack of oxygen in the tissues is sensed by the kidneys, which produce natural erythropoetin (EPO). Erythropoetin stimulates the bone marrow to produce more red blood cells.

EPO AND PERFORMANCE

Some athletes have taken synthetic EPO to enhance performance. But EPO is a banned substance. Although it may improve performance, it also increases the thickness of blood and is associated with an increased risk of stroke, heart attack, and death. These risks are great, making EPO very dangerous.

Some of the factors that may deprive the tissues of oxygen include blood loss due to bleeding, destruction of the bone marrow by radiation, high altitude, diseases that slow the circulation of blood to the tissues, and exercise. All these conditions result in increased production of red blood cells by normal bone marrow.

Androgens, or "male" hormones, are found in both men and women. Testosterone is the most important "male" hormone. Red blood cell production is increased in response to androgens. The much higher levels of androgens found in men contribute to the increased production of red blood cells in post-pubertal males. This is one reason why men have hemoglobin levels about 10% greater than those in women.

THE ROLE OF IRON

Iron is important in the formation of hemoglobin. About 65% of the iron in the body is in the form of hemoglobin. Storage iron, or ferritin, makes up about 25% of the iron in the body. Myoglobin, an iron-containing compound found in muscles, makes up about 4% of the iron in the body.

The average amount of iron in the body is about 4 grams. Men lose about 0.6 milligrams daily in the stool. Women lose about 2 milligrams daily, the increased average daily loss being due to the loss of blood during menstruation.

FOLIC ACID AND VITAMIN B_{12}

Folic acid and vitamin B_{12} are needed to produce red blood cells. A deficiency of either results in a reduced number of red blood cells and red blood cells that are larger than normal.

How Red Blood Cells Are Destroyed

Normal red blood cells have an average life of 120 days. Abnormalities in their size or shape are sensed by the spleen. The spleen acts as a filter, removing old or deformed red blood cells from the circulation. If red blood cells are not properly formed, they usually do not last as long as 120 days. Even if an average number of red blood cells are produced, abnormalities in their formation may also lead to anemia.

Causes of Anemia in the Athlete

"SPORTS" ANEMIA

Sports anemia is not related to iron deficiency. It's usually discovered on a routine blood test. The athlete has no symptoms.

Many athletes have an increased volume of blood. The total number of red blood cells present in the circulation of an athlete may be normal (or mildly increased). As the volume of blood is relatively higher, the concentration of red blood cells is actually reduced. The total oxygen-carrying capacity of the circulation is unchanged (or increased). This is athletic physiologic anemia and does not represent disease.

Figure 5-1

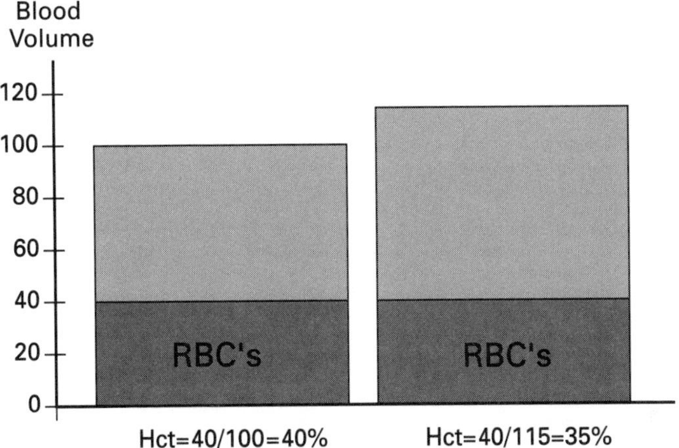

Physiologic anemia

Suppose the hematocrit—the percentage of red blood cells—is 40%. If the number of red blood cells remains the same, and the volume of the circulation increases 15%, the percentage of red blood cells will fall to 35%.

In some elite athletes, the high volume and the intensity of exercise reduces testosterone production. Since one of testosterone's actions is to increase red blood cell production, decreased testosterone may also contribute to sports anemia.

BLOOD LOSS ANEMIA

If you bleed from injury or blood donation, you'll be anemic until the body can replace your red blood cells. Assuming you lose a pint of blood, it will take about six weeks to replace it if you have all the building blocks for blood.

IRON-DEFICIENCY ANEMIA

This is the most common medical cause of anemia. Iron deficiency usually results from loss of iron in blood greater than that replaced by diet.

Women with heavy periods are most prone to this type of anemia. Blood donors are also at risk for using up their iron stores. Since silent blood loss may result from causes such as bowel cancer or ulcer, it is important to look for a cause of bleeding if one is not readily apparent. When anemia is discovered, the amount of iron or ferritin in the blood can be measured. If these are low, iron deficiency is diagnosed. This type of anemia is usually corrected by obtaining extra iron from iron supplements. Ferrous sulfate, easily purchased at the grocery store or pharmacy, is the supplement most often used. Replacing lost iron may cure the anemia but will not solve an underlying problem such as gastrointestinal blood loss.

FOLIC ACID OR VITAMIN B_{12} DEFICIENCY

Deficiency of either one of these vitamins causes anemia. Folic acid deficiency is one of the most common vitamin deficiencies in athletes.

HORMONE-RELATED ANEMIAS

Decreased testosterone production that occurs due to aging in men, decreased thyroid function, kidney failure, liver problems, and alcoholism are all associated with anemia.

BONE MARROW PROBLEMS

Bone marrow disease related to radiation exposure, industrial chemicals, drugs, or cancer can cause anemia.

INCREASED DESTRUCTION OF RED BLOOD CELLS

Sickle cell anemia, thalassemia and other abnormalities of hemoglobin formation, immune problems, and a deficiency of the enzyme glucose-6-phosphate all result in the increased destruction of red blood cells.

Anemia Needs Evaluation

Anemia is a serious barrier to athletic performance. Although iron deficiency is the most common cause, it must not be automatically assumed that anemia is caused by iron deficiency. Proper medical diagnosis and the determination of any underlying causes will help correct the problem and optimize performance.

Respiratory Infections

We all get a cold or the flu every once in a while. We suffer minor and major health problems. When is it OK to ride, and when should one take time off the bike?

Commonsense Story

My first job as a physician was as a camp doctor to 750 kids in the Laurentian Mountains of Canada. The camp director told me that my most important duty was to decide who could go swimming.

I went to an excellent medical school—one of the top ten in the world. I had received excellent training in the care of patients with heart attacks, diabetes, serious pneumonia, broken bones. However, I had received no training on deciding when a kid could go swimming. After more than twenty years of medical practice, I haven't found any books or other authorities that delve into this question either.

That first day of camp, the first patient showed up, looking pretty miserable. I knew he didn't want to go swimming. I asked him, just to be sure. "Are you kidding?" he said. "Let me stay in the bunk." The second patient of my professional career also had the sniffles. She looked pretty perky. "Do you want to go swimming?" I asked. "Of course," she said, "I just wanted some of those red lozenges last year's doctor used to give out." And so it went. It was pretty easy to tell who should and who shouldn't go swimming after all. I just asked my patients.

It's the same way for me personally. Sometimes when I have a cold I feel like riding. Sometimes I don't.

General Advice

If you are honest with yourself, you can usually figure out what you should do. Lots of cyclists call me up to ask what they should do. I usually ask them what they think. They almost always know. If you want to ride but think maybe you shouldn't, try riding half the distance you think is reasonable. If you feel OK, complete the ride.

Anaerobic efforts are more difficult when you are ill with a respiratory infection. It's usually a good idea to severely reduce or avoid them.

Self-Treatment

Aspirin or acetaminophen helps aches and pains. Decongestants help stuffiness and runny noses. Be careful about using decongestants around the time of competition—they are banned when present over a certain amount.

Watch for Fever and Muscle Aches

If you have a fever, go easy, if you go at all. Fever is associated with considerably increased metabolic demands on the body. Muscle aches sometimes are associated with potentially more dangerous infections that may cause complications with the increased stress of training. If muscle aches are associated with your infection, rest is wise.

No Throat or Nose Symptoms?

If you have a fever, muscle aches, and no symptoms above the neck—no sore throat, no nose symptoms—watch out. Exercise may significantly worsen some virus-caused conditions that fit this description.

Yellow or Green Stuff

When the color of sputum or nasal discharge is yellow or green, it often signifies a bacterial infection. If this lasts more than a few days or is associated with fever, antibiotics may help.

Sleeping Hints

Can't Sleep? Sometimes It's Normal

We all have occasional difficulty sleeping. Hard efforts, especially in the evening, may make it difficult to fall asleep. Bicycle racers may have anxiety about their next day's performance. Sleeping in a strange hotel room also causes sleep difficulty for many. By developing good sleep habits, as discussed below, you will increase your chances for a good night's sleep even the night before an important race.

Medical Causes of Insomnia

The amount of sleep needed varies from person to person. There is no "correct amount," although studies do show that adults function best on at least eight hours a night. The quantity and quality of sleep often decrease with age. As we get into our sixties and older, naps are more common.

Alcohol is one of the biggest causes of sleep disturbance. Although small quantities taken occasionally may help sleep, almost all regular drinkers sleep poorly. Depression is a frequent cause of insomnia and daytime fatigue. Over-the-counter drugs—especially decongestants—frequently result in insomnia. Caffeine—found not only in coffee and colas but also in some over-the-counter pain formulas—interrupts sleep. Prescription drugs, including some beta-blockers used for high blood pressure, may cause interrupted sleep and nightmares. Appetite suppressants, including amphetamines, interrupt sleep. Rebound insomnia occurs after discontinuance of some medications, including sleeping pills.

Almost any medical illness—because of the discomfort, pain, anxiety or depression associated with disease—causes insomnia. Heartburn, frequent urination from an enlarged prostate, and untreated diabetes are specific medical causes of insomnia.

Develop Good Sleep Habits

Get in the habit of doing the same good things before going to bed at night. By developing a pre-bed ritual, you will train your body to expect to go to sleep at the right time. A warm bath or shower helps some. Relaxation techniques or reading can help others.

Try to go to bed and get up at the same time each day, including weekends. Stimulating activity before bed may interfere with getting to sleep. For example, if you use the bedroom for working, eating, or watching television, your alertness may rise and you may have some difficulty sleeping.

Your sleep may improve if you exercise in the late afternoon or early evening. Catnaps may be restorative for some, but avoid sleeping longer than one hour during the day.

Avoid drinking any fluids for several hours before bedtime. When you are traveling, meal patterns may be disrupted. Racers may eat later or drink more fluids than usual because restaurant waiters keep refilling their water glasses. Racers may wish to hydrate well, and their sleep may therefore be disrupted by the need to rise several times during the night to urinate.

Racer's Ideal Sleeping Position—Right Side

From a health point of view, the most common medical problem associated with sleeping is backache. Lying on your stomach is the worst position for your back. Lying on the back is better, especially with some pillows under your knees. The best position for the back is lying on the side. A pillow between the legs may help you keep comfortable in this position.

If you lie on your left side, your heart falls towards your chest wall. If you lie on your right side, your heart falls away from the chest wall and the heart's action is less noticeable. Most of the time it doesn't matter whether you sleep on your left or your right side. But if you've raced the track at night, you know how your heart can pound for hours afterward. And if you are anxious about the next day's race, your heart action is more noticeable.

By learning to sleep on your right side, you'll be less bothered by the beating of your heart and more able to sleep. By learning to sleep on your right side—by training this way—you'll be able to sleep in this familiar best position the night before the big race.

Dealing with Light and Noise

Maybe your own bedroom is quiet and dark. But hotel rooms may be noisy and the drapes imperfect at keeping out the dawn's early light. By developing a ritual of sleeping with earplugs and blindfold, you'll be more impervious to the vagaries of your hotel room. If you use earplugs only rarely, the novelty of using them may decrease your chances for a good night's sleep. If you have trained yourself to use them, they can give you a great sleep when otherwise you might not get one. Turning the air conditioner on—even if it isn't so hot that you need it—may provide a low-level background noise that masks otherwise more disturbing sounds.

Sleeping Pills

The party line is that sleeping pills are "bad" and that "natural" therapies should be prescribed. When sleep is a problem, the placebo effect of any pill is strong. Almost all authorities agree that pharmacologically active sleeping pills, used on a regular basis, are a bad idea. Still, the need for a good night's sleep before an important event occasionally prompts some of us to reach for an artificial aid.

Melatonin, an over-the-counter sleeping aid, helps some people, but the long-term side effects are unknown and, as with many drugs not regulated by the F.D.A., formulation consistency and purity may be a problem. Some antihistamines, used for allergies, also cause drowsiness. This side effect is commonly exploited to aid sleep. Triazolam (Halcion) and zolpidem tartrate (Ambien) are short-acting agents currently popular with elite-level racers, but withdrawal symptoms, including rebound insomnia and other problems, plague users of sleeping pills.

Sleep—Train Specifically

Specific rituals and training help you perform better when needed. If the night before the big race is the first time you've slept in a hotel room all year, you may not sleep so well. The first night's sleep before a race in the new season is often the most difficult. The more you race and the more you sleep in hotel rooms, the easier it will be. Some tricks, such as using earplugs and a blindfold and learning to sleep on your right side, are specifically useful for racers. Good sleep habits can benefit us all!

Tetanus Shots

What We're Talking About

Commonly called lockjaw, tetanus is an uncommon but serious infection. Infection usually results from wound contamination with infectious spores. Infected spores in dust and soil are more common in warmer climates and in cultivated areas.

Who Should Get the Shot?

Routine booster shots are recommended for everyone. Since tetanus is more likely after a cut or scrape, and since skin injury is common in cyclists, all cyclists are encouraged to keep their immunization status current.

How Often

After childhood or other primary immunization, maintain your immunity with a booster dose once every ten years. Severe cuts, especially where tetanus spores are prevalent, may require a booster as soon as five years after the last one.

Flu Shots

Flu shots are not for everyone.

Flu Shots Prevent Influenza

The "flu shot" is a vaccine designed to prevent influenza type A. Influenza is an acute respiratory illness caused by infection with an influenza virus. The illness affects the upper and/or lower respiratory tracts and is often associated with fever, headache, muscle aches, and weakness. Outbreaks occur almost every year in the winter.

Types of Influenza Virus

There are three types of influenza virus: types A, B, and C. Most of the severe and extensive illness is associated with type A. Influenza virus changes every year. Sometimes the changes are small, sometimes large. When the changes are large, the annual winter epidemic is worse.

Vaccine Effectiveness

The pharmaceutical manufacturers anticipate the changes in the influenza virus by noting worldwide trends so as to more effectively prepare the next year's vaccine. When they guess right, the vaccine is 50% to 80% effective. When they guess wrong, the vaccine doesn't work well, and a lot more people get sick.

Side Effects

Vaccines are highly purified and are associated with few side effects. About 5% of patients will experience low-grade fever and mild flu-like symptoms eight to twenty-four hours after vaccination. Up to one-third may have redness or tenderness at the vaccination site. The vaccine is produced in eggs; individuals with egg allergy should not receive the vaccine.

When Should You Get Vaccinated?

The flu season is from December to March. Occasional outbreaks are a little earlier or later. The vaccine begins to work in a little more than a week. The vaccine's effectiveness is temporary; it wanes several months later. The timing of vaccination is generally early November. It's a trade-off. Get vaccinated too late, and you risk getting influenza early in the season. Get vaccinated too early, and you may not be well protected later in the flu season.

Who Should Get the Vaccine?

The U.S. Public Health Service recommends influenza vaccination for those at risk for complications of influenza. They include individuals with chronic heart or lung disease, residents of nursing homes and other chronic care facilities, those over 65, those who have required medical attention for diabetes or kidney disease, those with immune problems such as HIV, and those with blood problems such as sickle cell anemia. Individuals who come in contact with such patients are also advised to be vaccinated to prevent those at risk from coming in contact with influenza.

Not All Respiratory Illness Is the Flu

The vaccine helps prevent influenza, but not all respiratory winter illness is influenza. Most of the time it's a regular cold. Both the cold and the flu are associated with sore throat and nasal symptoms. Influenza is the more serious illness, associated with higher fever and more aches and pains.

Why Shouldn't You Get the Shot?

For those at risk of influenza complications now, it's probably better to get protection now. But if you are otherwise healthy, an argument can be made for you to forgo flu shots and develop natural immunity. When you get sick with influenza, the body builds up a natural immunity that lasts many years or decades. You remain protected, or partially protected, for years. This may help protect you from serious illness or complications later in life. If you start vaccines now, you won't develop the stronger, more permanent, natural immunity. Even with continued vaccination—if the pharmaceutical manufacturers guess wrong in their choice of parts for the vaccine—you may be more at risk for serious illness later in life.

High Blood Pressure Medicines

What We're Talking About

High blood pressure, or hypertension, is a common medical condition. Usually there are no symptoms, and most people don't know they have it until their blood pressure is checked. Most of the time there is no known cause.

It's normal for blood pressure to vary from doctor visit to doctor visit. In fact, it's normal for blood pressure to vary minute to minute. What counts in the diagnosis of hypertension is a blood pressure that remains consistently high.

Treatment

Hypertension may be initially treated with salt restriction, alcohol restriction, weight reduction, and exercise. If these measures are not successful, there are many effective medicines to treat this problem.

The main reason this chapter appears in this book is to alert you that at least three classes of high blood pressure medicines—diuretics, beta-blockers, and calcium-channel blockers—may interfere with athletic performance.

Diuretics, or "water pills," are good medicines for high blood pressure. They are often the first medicines selected in the treatment of hypertension. They are cheap, effective and usually need to be taken only once a day. Unfortunately, diuretics make you more prone to dehydration and so interfere with performance.

Beta-blockers are also a common class of medicines used in the treatment of high blood pressure. They too are effective, have few side effects, and are relatively inexpensive. Many need to be taken only once a day. Beta-blockers are also used to treat heart disease, to prevent migraine, and to reduce stage fright or performance anxiety. They limit the workload that the heart can accomplish. This can be an extremely important benefit in heart disease. Beta-blockers are, however, lousy for the performance athlete. If they are used effectively for medical disease, you often can't raise your heart rate to anaerobic threshold levels or beyond.

Calcium-channel blockers may limit the heart rate or reduce the force of contraction of the heart. This is especially true of verapamil (Calan, Isoptin). This may be a problem for some athletes.

Angiotensin-converting enzyme (ACE) inhibitors are first-line antihypertension medications, which are the least likely to interfere with athletic performance. Unfortunately, they are relatively expensive

Alert your doctor and find an antihypertension medicine suitable for athletes.

Hints for Kids and Juniors

Kids of any age need helmets just like everyone else. A baby can't support its head until 8 months or so. Many question the wisdom of lugging a child around in a bicycle trailer before that age. The use of a trailer makes the bicycle less responsive and more unstable. Lugging your kids around can help endurance and power, but it's not a time for speedwork, which might endanger you both. Have a few safe toys in the trailer with your kid. Stop at least every half hour. Most kids have a tough time if you ride more than a few hours total.

Children often don't anticipate environmental effects, including heat loss and sunburn. They need supervision.

Kids can ride "for fun" whenever they like, but children under the age of 8 are not ready for serious training. A child of eight might build up to a ride of about 10 miles. Hills, headwinds, or rain make distances seem much longer. Kids' bikes are not as efficient as adult bikes—the effort the rider needs to give is proportionally much larger.

Serious racing is not appropriate until a child is at least 10—some would say 12. Racing must always be fun. Pressure to compete, if any, must be self-generated. For many coaches, an important task is to protect children from overzealous adults. Go along with the desires of your child if they seem appropriate, but make sure you are not projecting your own desires onto your kid.

Structured rides for juniors are available in most cities with velodromes. Many local bicycle clubs have sections for junior riders. Junior riders develop best when competing against other riders of similar physical development. Sometimes this may be an older or a younger rider. There can be an enormous difference in physical maturity between a small-for-age rider racing against another rider just one year older who is big-for-age.

Good junior riders aged 15 and 16 may be able to compete with older riders of the lower categories. The best 17- and 18-year-old juniors are able to compete with local Cat 1 and 2 riders. Juniors are rarely competitive with older elite racers at bigger regional and national races, long races, and stage races.

Weight training for riders who have not achieved physical maturity is controversial and has some risks. Muscles are frequently stronger than developing bones, and overuse injuries can easily occur. Calisthenics or high-rep work is more appropriate than low-rep high-intensity work.

Big gears are thought to be harmful to a junior's short-term health and long-term development. Many junior races have gear restrictions underlining this concept.

Collegiate racing is a separate racing scene and is licensed and operated in conjunction with USA Cycling.

Bicycling for the Over-50-Year-Old

Although declines in performance occur with age, the majority of studies that measure performance find that most of the decline is due to a lower quality and quantity of training, injuries, and disease rather than to the effects of aging per se.

A general physical exam and treadmill electrocardiogram are often recommended for those over the age of 50 who want to begin any exercise program. Start exercising slowly, and if you don't have any problems, increase your activity level no more than 10% a week.

If you have the money, invest in a lightweight bicycle. They are more fun to ride because they respond more quickly to your efforts and allow you to keep up with others more easily.

If you are interested in fitness riding or competitive riding, know that the training principles that apply to Olympic competitors are the same principles that apply to riders of any age. The principal difference is that older riders are capable of a smaller volume, or quantity, of work.

Don't believe the conventional wisdom. Conventional wisdom applies to the population as a whole, not necessarily to you. For example, your maximum heart rate is probably not 220 minus your age—just as your height is probably not 5 feet 8 inches—even though that may be a population average.

Older riders often take longer to recover than younger riders. They also have more difficulty regaining fitness once they've lost it with a layoff. "If you don't use it, you lose it" applies even more to older riders than to younger ones.

Many older riders increase their enjoyment by joining a group of people of similar ages. Some are a little hesitant about joining a seniors' cycling group, thinking that they don't want to hear discussions about arthritis pills and cataract surgery. On the other hand, are you really interested in discussions of acne?

Glossary

ABDUCTION: Movement away from the midline of the body, as opposed to adduction.

ABRASION: Skin injury from friction. Road rash is a specific form of abrasion, usually caused by a fall or crash. Mild injury may result only in redness. More serious injury rubs away deep layers of skin and results in permanent scarring. Bicycle seat friction may also cause abrasions of the rear end, or crotch.

ACUTE: As a medical term, of recent or sudden onset or of short duration.

ADDUCTION: Movement toward the midline of the body, as opposed to abduction.

AEROBIC: Using oxygen with a fuel source. Implied intensity is below anaerobic level. Implied level of work is low enough so that buildup of lactic acid is avoided and exercise can be continued for prolonged periods.

AEROBIC CAPACITY: The maximum capability to produce aerobic work. VO_2 max is a synonym.

AERODYNAMIC: Reducing air resistance.

ANAEROBIC: Work without the presence of oxygen. Implies a high level of work intensity that can be maintained only for relatively short periods of time. A very short energy production system—that of creatine phosphate—can supply energy needs for about ten seconds without the production of lactic acid. Other anaerobic efforts result in higher levels of lactic acid.

ANAEROBIC THRESHOLD: That point at which work intensity results in an increasing anaerobic contribution. Defined differently depending upon the anaerobic marker used. The chapter "Thresholds" (see page 85) explains the details.

ANTI-INFLAMMATORY: Against inflammation.

ARTHRITIS: Inflammation of one or more joints. The usual cause is degeneration, or related to aging. Arthritis can also be caused by infection, injury, or immune or crystal deposits.

ATP: Adenosine triphosphate, a chemical in cells serving as an immediate source of energy. It is formed in the mitochondria.

ATROPHY: To decrease in size. Often used in reference to muscle cells, which decrease in size with disuse or decreased training.

BIG GEARS: Bicycle gears requiring a large amount of force to turn.

BLOW-UP: Go out too fast and be unable to continue.

BONK: Run out of energy, tire. Usually implies glycogen depletion.

BRUISE: The leakage of blood around muscle or under tissues as a result of direct trauma. The medical term is *contusion*.

BURSITIS: Inflammation of a bursa, a cystic structure that forms between two surfaces that move over each other, often lubricating that movement.

CADENCE: Revolutions per minute of pedal stroke.

CAPILLARY: Tiniest blood vessel, located between the arterial and venous systems.

CARBOHYDRATE LOADING: A dietary procedure resulting in increased muscle glycogen.

CARDIORESPIRATORY: Referring to the heart and lungs.

CARDIOVASCULAR: Referring to the heart and blood vessels.

CHONDROMALACIA: A weakening or softening of bone. Most commonly the kneecap is affected.

CHRONIC: As a medical term, of long duration.

CONCENTRIC: As a weight-training term, refers to when the muscle contracts and shortens, as opposed to an eccentric contraction. When you raise yourself to a chin-up, the muscle is contracting concentrically.

CONTUSION: A bruise. The leakage of blood around muscle or under tissues as a result of direct trauma.

CRAMP: A painful, localized temporary spasm of muscle.

CREATINE PHOSPHATE: A chemical in cells that can briefly replenish ATP and thereby produce energy for very short (up to ten-second) events.

DEGENERATIVE ARTHRITIS: Degeneration of joint surfaces, and the consequences that result from wear and tear or previous trauma.

DISLOCATION: An injury that displaces the joint surfaces out of position. There is also some damage to the ligaments around the joint, and sometimes a fracture as well.

DROP: The lower part of a road handlebar. Also, to ride faster and away from another rider or group.

DURATION: Length of time spent performing an interval. If work is continuous, volume and duration are the same.

ECCENTRIC: As a weight-training term, refers to when the muscle contracts and lengthens, as opposed to a concentric contraction. When you let yourself down slowly from a chin-up, the muscle is contracting eccentrically.

ENDURANCE: Ability to last.

ENERGY: The capacity to perform work.

ERGOGENIC: Special substances or treatments used to improve physiological, psychological, or biomechanical function. They may include nutritional, pharmacological, or psychological approaches.

EXTENSION: Straightening out of a body part. Movement of a joint so that the two parts of it are placed farther apart. The opposite of flexion.

FARTLEK: "Speed play," unstructured intervals.

FAST TWITCH: Muscle fiber type characterized by a fast response to nerve stimulation. This type of muscle fiber tends to be useful in strength or power activities such as sprinting.

FATIGUE: The inability to maintain a level of work.

FLEXIBILITY: The range of motion of the body's joints.

FLEXION: Bending in of a body part. Movement of a joint so that the two parts of it are placed closer together. The opposite of extension.

FREE WEIGHTS: Weights not part of an exercise machine.

GLUCOSE: A simple sugar, used by the body for energy.

GLYCEROL: A three-carbon chain molecule. It forms the backbone of triglycerides.

GLYCOGEN: A complex sugar. A form of storage energy in the body.

GROWTH HORMONE: A pituitary hormone involved in growth and development.

HAMMER: Hard sustained effort.

HAMSTRINGS: Muscles in the back of the thigh.

HYPERTROPHY: Increase in size. Often used in reference to muscle cells, which increase in size, rather than in number, in response to training.

INFLAMMATION: A process consisting of body reactions to an injury or situation caused by physical, chemical, or biological agents. It may include redness, heat, swelling, pain, or loss of function. Local reactions and responses lead to repair and healing.

INTENSITY: Load or speed of work.

INTERVAL: Period of hard work. On the bicycle, a period of riding hard.

ISOKINETIC: In weight training, related to a muscle contraction in which load changes with muscle movement. Muscles can produce different amounts of force through their range of motion. Nautilus, Cybex, and other machines are designed to accommodate this changing strength. See *isometric* and *isotonic.*

ISOMETRIC: In weight training, refers to a muscle contraction with little or no joint movement. For example, a quadriceps isometric exercise is to straighten the leg and then tighten the quad without moving the knee. See *isokinetic* and *isotonic.*

ISOTONIC: In weight training, refers to a muscle contraction in which load does not change with muscle movement. This is the type of weight training provided by dumbbells and barbells. See *isokinetic* and *isometric.*

JAM: High-speed riding.

JOINT: A point of contact between bones.

JUMP: A short, quick burst of speed.

KICK: Final burst of speed.

LACTATE, LACTIC ACID: Products of the body's metabolism. Muscles produce lactic acid, which forms lactate in blood. Normally the blood contains less than 1.5 millimoles of lactate per liter. Depending upon the definition used, the anaerobic threshold is between 2 and 7 millimoles per liter. Levels higher than this cannot be sustained for prolonged periods of time.

LATERAL: The anatomical term meaning "away from the body." For general readability, we use the term *outside*. Anatomists reserve the word *outside* for parts that encompass others (in as "the skull is outside the brain").

LEAN BODY MASS: Mass or weight without fat.

LEG SPEED: How fast one can turn the cranks.

LIGAMENT: A structure that connects bone to bone, usually around a joint.

LOWER EXTREMITY: Term for the hip, thigh, leg, ankle, and foot. The colloquial term *leg* is too imprecise. Medically speaking, the leg is the anatomical area between the thigh and the ankle.

MAXIMUM HEART RATE: The highest heart rate for a given person. In practical terms, the highest heart rate achieved by a rider within the past year. Session maximum heart rate is the highest heart rate achieved during a workout. Estimating your predicted maximum heart rate by subtracting your age from 220 is unreliable.

MEDIAL: The anatomical term meaning "toward the body." For general readability, we use the term *inside*. Anatomists reserve the word *inside* for parts that are encompassed by others (in as "the brain is inside the skull").

MITOCHONDRIA: The energy factories of cells, where the body produces adenosine triphosphate (ATP) by aerobic metabolism.

MUFFIN RIDE: Non-competitive supportive ride of friends with a muffin or pastry stop as a destination.

MUSCLE PULL OR STRAIN: A stretching injury to muscles. First-degree strains involve only excessive stretching, second-degree stains are partial tears, and third-degree strains are complete tears of muscles.

MUSCLE: A tissue that contracts to move or stabilize body parts.

NERVE COMPRESSION SYNDROME: The compression of a nerve, giving rise to pain and/or other neurological symptoms. Carpal tunnel and piriformis syndrome are examples.

NOODLE: To ride slowly.

NSAID: Non-steroidal anti-inflammatory drug. Medicines that reduce inflammation. They are available over the counter and by prescription. They do not contain cortisone or other steroid drugs.

OVER-TRAINING: Lack of fitness related to excessive intensity or duration of training. Can result from psychological or physical causes.

OVERUSE INJURY: A chronic, uncontrolled, overload, microtraumatic event. Overuse injuries occur over a period of time when forces applied to a structure are increased faster than the structure can adapt, or exceed its limits of adaptation.

OXYGEN DEBT: Amount of oxygen used by the body during a recovery period from a work or interval period that is in excess of that used with work.

PEAK: Good form, high physical fitness. Often the result of hard work combined with a period of good recovery.

PERIODIZATION: Training different aspects of fitness at different periods of time.

PERIOSTITIS: Inflammation of the periostium, the membrane covering the surface of bone. It is often caused by excessive pulling of ligaments or tendons that attach to it.

POWER: Work performed per unit of time. A combination of strength and speed.

QUADRICEPS: Muscle in the front of the thigh.

RATING OF PERCEIVED EXERTION (RPE): A subjective measure of intensity.

RECOVERY: The process of readying fitness systems to make further efforts. Period of training when one is not working hard. Rest is a type of recovery in which no activity takes place; active recovery includes light training.

REP, REPETITION: One rep is one complete movement of an exercise. Reps are the number of times a task or interval is repeated. See *set*.

RESTING HEART RATE: Heart rate at rest, popularly taken first thing in the morning, while one is still lying at rest in bed.

ROAD RASH: Skin abrasion, usually the result of a crash. Mild injury may result only in redness. More serious injury rubs away deep layers of skin and results in permanent scarring.

ROLLERS: Stationary training device with three cylindrical tubes (rollers) upon which a bicycle sits.

SEAT TUBE: Tube connecting the bottom bracket to the top tube.

SET: In training, a group of repetitions.

SLOW TWITCH: Muscle fiber type characterized by a slow response to nerve stimulation. This type of muscle fiber tends to be useful in endurance activities.

SMALL GEARS: Bicycle gears requiring a small amount of force to turn. Often used for recovery riding or to develop leg speed.

SNAP: The ability to accelerate quickly.

SPECIFICITY: Training principle stating that you specifically improve those characteristics of fitness that you train.

SPEED: Quickness, how fast one can go.

SPIN: Often used to mean high cadence, it more accurately refers to the fluidity or suppleness of the pedal stroke.

SPRAIN: A stretching injury to a ligament or group of ligaments. First-degree sprains involve only excessive stretching, second-degree sprains are partial tears, and third-degree strains are complete tears of ligaments.

STATIONARY TRAINER: Training device that does not move. Rollers, Lifecycles, Spinners, Turbo Trainers, and Trax stands are all varieties of stationary trainers.

STRAIN: A stretching injury to muscles. First-degree strains involve only excessive stretching, second-degree strains are partial tears, and third-degree strains are complete tears of muscles.

STRENGTH: Force that can be applied. Muscular strength is the greatest amount of force that can be produced in a single maximal effort.

STRESS FRACTURE: Weakened bone caused by excessive stress. If not properly rested, a stress fracture may progress to a complete fracture. Stress fractures are usually diagnosed by methods more sophisticated than regular X rays.

STRESS INJURY: A milder form and precursor of a stress fracture.

SUBLUXATION: An incomplete dislocation.

TACTIC: Action taken to further an overall strategy.

TENDONITIS: Inflammation of a tendon. A tendon connects muscle to bone.

TOP TUBE: In traditional bicycles, the horizontal tube connecting the steering column to the seat tube.

TRAINING AGE: The amount of time, usually in years, that an individual has been participating in a specific training program.

TRAINING CURVE: A curve, or graph, plotting aspects of fitness and time.

TRAINING EFFECT: The body's response and adaptation to physical demands.

TRAINING TRIANGLE: Training concept used to show the interdependence of several aspects of fitness in a visual plot.

TRAUMATIC INJURY: A sudden, or acute, injury. Lacerations (cuts), abrasions, and fractures are typical cycling traumatic injuries.

TURBO TRAINER: Brand name of a type of stationary trainer device.

UPPER EXTREMITY: Term for the shoulder, arm, forearm, wrist, and hand. The colloquial term *arm* is too imprecise. Medically speaking, the arm is the anatomical area between the shoulder and the forearm.

VO_2 MAX: The maximum uptake of oxygen a person can utilize to produce energy. A measure of the ability of muscles to use oxygen. An important determinant of fitness and success.

VOLUME OF TRAINING: Total time of intense training. If training is continuous, volume and duration are the same.

Selected References

Baker, Arnie. *Smart Cycling—Training and Racing for Riders of All Levels.* New York: Simon & Schuster, 1997.

Bartok-Oslon, C. J., et al. "Prevalence of Eating Disorder Symptoms in Female Collegiate College Cyclists." *Medicine & Science in Sports & Exercise* Suppl. Vol. 28, No. 5, May 1996.

Birnbaum, Jacob S. *The Musculoskeletal Manual.* Orlando Fla.: Grune & Stratton, 1986.

Borysewicz, Edward. *Bicycle Road Racing.* Brattleboro, Vt.: Vitess Press, 1985.

Brechtel, L. M., et al. "Non-Responding of the Sympathoadrenal System—a Diagnostic Sign for the Overtraining Syndrome." *Medicine & Science in Sports and Exercise* Suppl. Vol. 28 No. 5, May 1996.

Burke, Edmund. *Science of Cycling.* Champaign, Ill.: Human Kinetics Books, 1986.

Chryssanthopoulus, C. "Influence of a Pre-Exercise Meal and a Carbohydrate Electrolyte Solution on Endurance Running Capacity." *Medicine & Science in Sports & Exercise* Suppl. Vol. 28, No. 5, May 1996.

Coleman, Ellen. "Sports Drink Update." *Sports Science Exchange* No. 5, http://www.gssiweb.com, 1988.

Coyle, Edward. "Fat Metabolism During Exercise." *Sports Science Exchange* No. 59, http://www.gssiweb.com, 1995.

Crowley, M. A., et al. "Effects of Cycling Cadence on VO_2 Kinetics and Delta Efficiency. *Medicine & Science in Sports & Exercise* Suppl. Vol. 28, No. 5, May 1996.

Derman, K. D., et al. "Fuel Kinetics During Intense Running and Cycling in Triathletes Ingesting Carbohydrate." *Medicine & Science in Sports & Exercise* Suppl. Vol. 28, No. 5, May 1996.

Eichner, E. R., Ergolytic Drugs, *Sports Science Exchange* No. 15, http://www.gssiweb.com, 1989.

———, et al. "Hyponatremia in Sport: Symptoms and Prevention." *Sports Science Exchange Roundtable* No. 12, http://www.gssiweb.com, 1993.

———, et al. "The Kidney, Exercise, and Hydration." *Sports Science Exchange Roundtable* No. 17, http://www.gssiweb.com, 1994.

Fuentes, Robert. "Nutritional Ergogenic Aids." *Helix Education*, http://www.helix.com, 1996.

Garrick, James, and David Webb. *Sports Injuries, Diagnosis and Management.* Philadelphia: W. B. Saunders, 1990.

Gisolfi, Carl. "Exercise, Intestinal Absorption, and Rehydration." *Sports Science Exchange* No. 32, http://www.gssiweb.com, 1991.

———, et al. "Intestinal Fluid Absorption in Exercise and Disease." *Sports Science Exchange Roundtable* No. 11, http://www.gssiweb.com, 1993.

Gulledge, T. P., et al. "Reproducibility of Low Resting Testosterone Levels in Endurance Trained Men." *Medicine & Science in Sports & Exercise* Suppl. Vol. 28, No. 5, May 1996.

Guyton, Arthur. *Textbook of Medical Physiology. Philadelphia:* W. B. Saunders, 1996.

Hawley, J. A., et al. "Effect of Ingesting Varying Concentrations of Sodium on Fluid Balance during Exercise." *Medicine & Science in Sports & Exercise* Suppl. Vol. 28, No. 5, May 1996.

Heath, E. M., et al. "Effect of Niacin on Endurance Performance in Cyclists." *Medicine & Science in Sports & Exercise* Suppl. Vol. 28, No. 5, May 1996.

Heil, D. P. "Theoretical Hip and Knee Extensor Torques as a Function of Preferred Hip Angle and Crank Angle in Cyclists." *Medicine & Science in Sports & Exercise* Suppl. Vol. 28, No. 5, May 1996.

Hotell, M. D., et al. "Carbohydrate Paste Ingestion during Prolonged Treadmill Running." *Medicine & Science in Sports & Exercise* Suppl. Vol. 28, No. 5, May 1996.

Hyatt, J. P., et al. "Exercise-Induced Muscle Damage in Subjects with Different Levels of Ingested Estrogen." *Medicine & Science in Sports & Exercise* Suppl. Vol. 28, No. 5, May 1996.

Janssen, Peter G. J. M., *Training, Lactate, Pulse.* Oulu, Finland: Polar Electro Oy, 1987.

Krebs, P. S. "Effects of Varying Bicycle Crank Length on Exercise VO_2 Response." *Medicine & Science in Sports & Exercise* Suppl. Vol. 28, No. 5, May 1996.

Kreider R., et al. "Effects of Ingesting a Lean Mass Promoting Supplement During Resistance Training on Isokinetic Performance." *Medicine & Science in Sports & Exercise* Suppl. Vol. 28, No. 5, May 1996.

Lamb, David R. *Physiology of Exercise—Responses and Adaptations.* New York: Macmillan, 1984.

Levine, B. D., et al. "Confirmation of the "High-Low" Hypothesis: Living at Altitude—Training Near Sea Level Improves Sea Level Performance." *Medicine & Science in Sports & Exercise* Suppl. Vol. 28, No. 5, May 1996.

Manjra, S., et al. "Risk Factors for Exercise Associated Muscle Cramping." *Medicine & Science in Sports & Exercise* Suppl. Vol. 28, No. 5, May 1996.

Matheny, Fred. *Weight Training for Cyclists.* Brattleboro, Vt.: Velo-news, 1986.

Maughen, Ronald, and Nancy Rehrer. "Gastric Emptying During Exercise." *Sports Science Exchange* No. 46, http://www.gssiweb.com, 1993.

Maughen, Ronald, et al. "Rehydration and Recovery After Exercise." *Sports Science Exchange* No. 62, http://www.gssiweb.com, 1996.

McArdle, William, Frank Katch, and Victor Katch. *Exercise Physiology.* Philadelphia: Lea & Feiberger, 1994.

Mellion, Morris B., and Edmund Burke. "Bicycling Injuries." *Clinics in Sports Medicine.* Philadelphia: W. B. Saunders, 1994.

Millar, A. L., et al. "The Effects of Massage on Delayed Onset Muscle Soreness, Force Production and Physiological Parameters." *Medicine & Science in Sports & Exercise* Suppl. Vol. 28, No. 5, May 1996.

Murray, Bob. "Fluid Replacement: The American College of Sports Medicine Position Stand." *Science Exchange* No. 63, http://www.gssiweb.com, 1996.

Myburgh, K. H., et al. "Creatine Supplementation and Sprint Training in Cyclists:

Metabolic and Performance Effects." *Medicine & Science in Sports & Exercise* Suppl. Vol. 28, No. 5, May 1996.

Nemoto, I. "Branched-Chain Amino Acid Supplementation Improves Endurance Capacities and RPE." *Medicine & Science in Sports & Exercise* Suppl. Vol. 28, No. 5, May 1996.

O'Toole, M. L. "Daily Vitamin E Supplementation Prior to Ultraendurance Exercise." *Medicine & Science in Sports & Exercise* Suppl. Vol. 28, No. 5, May 1996.

Pearl, Bill. "Getting Stronger." Bolinas, Calif.: Shelter Publications, 1986.

Perez, H. R., et al. "The Effects of Chromium Nicotinamide on Body Composition and Resting BMR of Sedentary Females." *Medicine & Science in Sports & Exercise* Suppl. Vol. 28, No. 5, May 1996.

Roy, Karen, and Thurlow Rogers. *Fit & Fast*. Brattleboro, Vt.: Vitess Press, 1989.

Schirmer, G. P., et al. "Vitamin and Mineral Status of Trained Competitive Cyclists during One Year of Training." *Medicine & Science in Sports & Exercise* Suppl. Vol. 28, No. 5, May 1996.

Sherman, William. "Exercise and Type I Diabetes." *Sports Science Exchange* No. 25, http://www.gssiweb.com, 1990.

———. "Exercise and Type II Diabetes." *Sports Science Exchange* No. 37, http://www.gssiweb.com, 1992.

Sutton, John. "Exercise Training at High Altitude: Does It Improve Endurance Performance at Sea Level." *Sports Science Exchange* No. 45, http://www.gssiweb.com, 1993.

Terrados, N., et al. "Hormonal Changes during a Professional Cycling Road Race." *Medicine & Science in Sports & Exercise* Suppl. Vol. 28, No. 5, May 1996.

Terrillion, K. A., et al. "The Effect of Creatine Supplementation on Two 700-M Maximal Running Bouts." *Medicine & Science in Sports & Exercise* Suppl. Vol. 28, No. 5, May 1996.

Tidus, P. M. "Endurance Training Does Not Affect Glutathione or Vitamin E Status in Human Muscle." *Medicine & Science in Sports & Exercise* Suppl. Vol. 28, No. 5, May 1996.

Voelz, J. "The Effects of High-Dose Ephedrine HCl on High-Intensity Treadmill Performance." *Medicine & Science in Sports & Exercise* Suppl. Vol. 28, No. 5, May 1996.

Wagenmakers, A. J. M., et al. "Carbohydrate Feedings Improve 1 Hour Time Trial Cycling Performance." *Medicine & Science in Sports & Exercise* Suppl. Vol. 28, No. 5, May 1996.

Walton, P. T. "The Effects of Pre-Exercise Carbohydrate Ingestion on Anaerobic Exercise." *Medicine & Science in Sports & Exercise* Suppl. Vol. 28, No. 5, May 1996.

Wilber, R. L., et al. "Comparison of Physiological Profiles of Elite Off-Road Cyclists and Elite Road Cyclists. *Medicine & Science in Sports & Exercise* Suppl. Vol. 28, No. 5, May 1996.

Williams, Melvin H. *Beyond Training*. Champaign, Ill.: Leisure Press, 1989.

Williamson, D., et al. "A Single Bout of Resistance Exercise Increases Basal Metabolic Rate in Healthy 60–70 Year Old Men." *Medicine & Science in Sports & Exercise* Suppl. Vol. 28, No. 5, May 1996.

Wilson, Jean D., et al. *Harrison's Textbook of Internal Medicine*. New York: McGraw-Hill, 1991.

INDEX

Numbers in italics indicate illustrations

About the Author

Dr. Arnie Baker is a licensed physician in San Diego, California. He obtained his M.D. as well as a master's degree in surgery from McGill University. He is a board-certified family practitioner. Before retiring to ride, coach, and write, he devoted approximately half of his medical practice to bicyclists. A bicycling-physician consultant, he serves on the fitness board of *Bicycling* magazine and is a medical consultant to USA Cycling.

He has authored six books and more than 500 articles on bicycling and bicycling-related subjects.

Arnie has been coaching since 1987. A professional, licensed USCF coach, he has coached racers to more than fifty U.S. National Championships and twenty U.S. records.

A racer as well as a coach, Arnie has a Category 1 USCF racing license. He has held five U.S. 40-K time trial records, has won multiple national championships, and has won more than 150 races. An all-around racer, he was the first to medal in every championship event in his district in a single year.

Active in the administration of the sport, he was USCF Western Sectional Masters Rep and Track Director of the San Diego Velodrome.

Arnie was President of Cyclo-Vets, his career cycling club, from 1987 to 1989, supervising its growth from 50 to 300 members and bringing the U.S. Masters National Championships to San Diego in 1990 and 1991. He was elected honorary President for life of Cyclo-Vets in 1990. He has helped lead his club to win the Masters Nationals Challenge Cup as the highest placed club at Nationals every year since the award came into existence.